100 Questions & Answers About HIV and AIDS

FIFTH EDITION

Paul E. Sax, MD

Clinical Director, Division of Infectious Diseases
Brigham and Women's Hospital
Professor of Medicine
Harvard Medical School
Boston, MA

JONES & BARTLETT
LEARNING

World Headquarters
Jones & Bartlett Learning
5 Wall Street
Burlington, MA 01803
978-443-5000
info@jblearning.com
www.jblearning.com

Jones & Bartlett Learning books and products are available through most bookstores and online booksellers. To contact Jones & Bartlett Learning directly, call 800-832-0034, fax 978-443-8000, or visit our website, www.jblearning.com.

Substantial discounts on bulk quantities of Jones & Bartlett Learning publications are available to corporations, professional associations, and other qualified organizations. For details and specific discount information, contact the special sales department at Jones & Bartlett Learning via the above contact information or send an email to specialsales@jblearning.com.

Production Credits

Product Manager: Joanna Gallant
Product Assistant: Melina Leon
Senior Project Specialist: Dan Stone
Digital Project Specialist: Angela Dooley
Director of Marketing: Andrea DeFronzo
Marketing Manager: Lindsay White
Manufacturing and Inventory Control Supervisor: Wendy Kilborn
Composition: S4Carlisle Publishing Services
Cover Design: Scott Moden
Senior Media Development Editor: Troy Liston
Rights Specialist: John Rusk
Cover Images: Shutterstock/Charlotte Purdy; Shutterstock/Nadasaki; Shutterstock/Kiselev Andrey Valerevich
Printing and Binding: CJK Group Inc.

ISBN: 978-1-284-20073-7

6048

Printed in the United States of America
24 23 22 21 20   10 9 8 7 6 5 4 3 2 1

Contents

Foreword

Nearly 40 years into the HIV epidemic, there is an enormous amount of information available for both patients and clinicians on HIV and AIDS. With websites and textbooks and pamphlets galore, one would wonder if there is a need for another book about AIDS. I would argue that now, more than ever, we need to help our patients find answers to all of their questions about preventing and living with HIV. With such an abundance of information, there is never enough time to figure out what information is both clear and reliable. *100 Questions & Answers About HIV and AIDS, Fifth Edition*, delivers on both these measures. It is a tremendous resource for people living with HIV, as well as their friends, family members, and healthcare providers.

Judith Currier, MD
Professor of Medicine
Chief, Division of Infectious Diseases
Co-Director, UCLA Center for
Clinical AIDS Research and Education
David Geffen School of Medicine at
University of California, Los Angeles

Introduction and Preface to the Fifth Edition

My motivation to become an HIV specialist began during my medical internship in 1987. HIV was rapidly becoming the leading cause of death among young adults in the United States. There was both tremendous clinical need and terrible ongoing stigma—both for people with HIV and their clinicians. Despite these challenges, the people we cared for demonstrated extraordinary hope, remarkable courage, and—perhaps most amazingly, given our limited treatments—wonderful gratitude to their care providers.

Fortunately, HIV treatment took a huge leap forward in the mid-1990s, when combination antiretroviral therapy (ART) rapidly became standard of care. As noted in the first chapter of this book, a person with HIV on treatment can expect to live as long as someone who doesn't have HIV. This is truly one of the most extraordinary advances in the history of medicine!

When someone contacted me last year about revising Joel Gallant's book, *100 Questions & Answers About HIV and AIDS*, I confess I had some trepidation. A good friend of mine, Joel is also a brilliant teacher and a gifted writer—so how could I improve on perfection? A glance through the latest editions of the book confirmed my impressions, so I've taken the liberty (with his permission) of retaining much of what he's written. I've provided necessary updates, added my own personal anecdotes, and inserted my voice (and jokes) periodically. But this is still Joel's creation, and I thank him for the opportunity to contribute to it.

Paul E. Sax, MD

PART ONE

Now That You Know

What's my prognosis?

Can I live a normal life?

What about sex and relationships?

Who should I tell?

More . . .

1. What's my prognosis?

"Prognosis" is the medical term for how we doctors and other clinicians expect an illness to turn out. And the good news is that your prognosis is excellent! HIV does not mean a progressive, fatal illness anymore—those were the bad old days. The memory of those horrible times, together with the stigma that still surrounds HIV, can make learning you have HIV a lot harder than it should be. With the right treatment, HIV is a manageable disease. If it didn't come with so much emotional, social, and historical baggage, people would react to the diagnosis the way they might if they learned that they had high blood pressure, diabetes, or arthritis. Granted, these aren't perfect examples because you can't transmit these problems to others, but they share with HIV the fact that they are lifelong conditions that require ongoing treatment. On the other hand, treatment for HIV is far easier and more effective than treatment for any of these diseases!

Antiretroviral therapy (ART) is the term we use to describe the medications that stop the **virus** from replicating (multiplying or reproducing). When referring to "therapy" in this book, I'm referring to ART. Other terms you'll sometimes hear are **highly active antiretroviral therapy (abbreviated HAART)**, **combination antiretroviral therapy (cART)**, and **cocktail** terms coined to distinguish combination therapy from the less effective treatment we used in the 1980s and early 1990s. Pet peeve alert—I don't like the terms "HAART" and "cocktail"; they are very outdated! (And if you're going to have a "cocktail", why not have the real kind? Provided, of course, it's in moderation.) The bottom line is that since *all* HIV treatment is now HAART and cART, and has been for over two decades, it's easier and more accurate just to use the term "ART."

Antiretroviral therapy (ART)

Drug therapy that stops HIV from replicating and improves the function of the immune system.

Virus

A microscopic organism composed of genetic material (DNA or RNA) inside a protein coat.

Highly active antiretroviral therapy (HAART)

Antiretroviral therapy meant to suppress the viral load to undetectable levels, using a combination of several drugs to prevent resistance. Since all HIV treatment has been combination therapy for more than two decades, now we just refer to it as antiretroviral therapy (ART).

Combination antiretroviral therapy (cART)

Another term for "HAART"—still sometimes used in research papers.

Cocktail

An outdated term for an antiretroviral regimen (a combination of antiretroviral drugs). Let's stop using this term!

By stopping the **replication** of HIV, ART protects the **immune system**—the system in the body that fights infections and cancers—keeping it from being damaged and allowing it to recover. The development of ART is up there with the discovery of antibiotics and vaccines as one of the greatest medical achievements of all time—and treatment keeps getting better!

ART has completely changed the outlook for people with HIV. There is no time limit to the benefits of therapy once you start. If you take your medications faithfully, you can keep HIV in control for life—a *long* life—having to change therapy only because of side effects or because better drugs come along.

If you've just been diagnosed, plan on sticking around for a long time, living long enough to die of old age. There is no need to change your life plans based on your diagnosis.

If you start ART and take it faithfully, you can probably live out a normal life span and die of old age. While we can't yet promise that the quality of your life will be exactly the same as it would have been if you didn't have HIV, I feel confident telling my patients that we can eliminate the possibility that they'll ever die of AIDS. This message especially applies to people who start therapy relatively soon after they acquire HIV and in those who have never had a weakened immune system from HIV.

> **Replication**
>
> The reproduction or multiplication of an organism, including HIV. The replication of HIV is a complex, multi-step process involving infection of a human cell and use of both viral enzymes and human cellular machinery to create new virus particles, which are then released and can infect new cells.

> **Immune system**
>
> The system in the body that fights infection and protects us from some cancers.

> *If you start ART early and take it faithfully, you can probably live out a normal life span and die of old age.*

2. Can I live a normal life? What about sex and relationships?

You *can* have a normal life, but it takes some commitments. Compared to someone with no chronic medical conditions, you'll have more medical visits and will take medications. However, treatment for HIV is now simple. Many of my patients now take just one pill once a day and see me for 30 minutes every 6 months; some are so reliable they check in annually. They're busy with work or school or family, travel, stay physically active, and maintain relationships.

The biggest adjustments are often the ones that have to do with your relationships with others. Friends and family members may have to be educated before they can treat you like they did before. Sexual relationships present a special challenge. Current partners, if they're negative, will have to face their own fear of infection—a fear not all relationships survive. Entering into new relationships involves the complex issues of **disclosure** and the fear of rejection or loss of confidence (Question 4).

Disclosure

The process of revealing your HIV status to others.

It may be hard to believe now, but in time, HIV will be low on your list of daily concerns, having little impact on the life you lead and the decisions you make. Getting to that point takes time, support, and sometimes counseling. You may feel overwhelmed now but stick with it … *it gets better*! Most of my patients say they rarely think about the fact that they have HIV. Taking their medications is a routine they barely notice, like brushing their teeth each day—only they usually only have to take their medications once a day and brush their teeth twice!

3. What do I do now?

Right after diagnosis, there are some important things you should do sooner than later. Keeping busy with constructive activities can help you cope with your new diagnosis.

- Notify your contacts: Anyone you had sex with should be notified so that they can get tested (Questions 4 and 85).

- Find an experienced HIV healthcare provider. Question 18 discusses how to find a provider who has expertise in treating HIV.

- Get some lab tests. The most important tests are the **CD4 count** (or **CD4 cell count**, sometimes called "T-cell count"), **viral load (plasma HIV RNA)**, and a **resistance test**, discussed in **Part 5**.

- Educate yourself. Reading this book is a good start, but don't stop here. You'll find more sources of information in the Appendix. There is a *ton* of information available for free online—I'll steer you to some of the best sites.

- Think about money. How are you going to pay for care? Do you have insurance? What does it cover? Do you qualify for any benefits on the basis of your HIV? If you're not sure, talk to a social worker or case manager (Question 21).

- Get support. Seek out the people in your life who you can talk to about having HIV, and tell them. If there aren't any, find a good counselor, therapist, or support group. Don't go through this alone (Question 4)!

CD4 count (or CD4 cell count)

A lab test that measures the number of CD4 cells in the blood (expressed as number of cells per cubic millimeter). It is sometimes referred to as the "T-helper count"—both terms mean the same thing. The CD4 count is the most important measure of the strength of your immune system, with higher numbers showing a stronger, healthier immune system. A normal count is more than 600 or so; most people don't get complications from HIV until the CD4 is less than 200. The CD4 cell count also tells you how urgent it is for you to start treatment.

4. Who should I tell?

Telling people about your HIV status is a big step, especially when you've just found out you're positive. Some people should be told right away, but with others you have time to think it over. Remember—there is no rush!

Viral load (or plasma HIV RNA)

A lab test that measures the amount of HIV in the plasma (blood), expressed as "copies per millimeter." The viral load predicts how fast your CD4 cell count will fall, with a faster decline seen with higher viral loads. It is the most important test for measuring the effectiveness of ART and assessing how likely you are to pass the virus on to another person through sexual contact.

Resistance test

A blood test that looks for HIV that is resistant to antiretroviral medications. The most commonly ordered test is called a "genotype," meaning that the lab looks at the genetic components of HIV to see if it is resistant.

It's important to tell sex partners or people you've shared needles with, because they could have given you HIV, or the other way around. They need to find out so they can get tested, for their own benefit and to protect others. Your provider, counselor, or case manager may also be able to help you inform partners. If those don't seem like good options, state health departments can notify your contacts and advise them to get tested without revealing your name.

Think about telling a friend or family member you rely on for emotional support. It's critical to have a solid support system. Think about the important people in your life. Will they be there for you? Will they respect your confidentiality? If so, consider telling them. But this is important—family members don't need to know just because they're family members. The same goes for friends. You pose no risk to them, and you may outlive them anyway. You should tell them if doing so will make you feel better, especially if they'll be part of your support network.

If you're not comfortable telling friends or family members, then you need to look elsewhere. Ask about support groups, counselors, peer advocates, or therapists in your community. While online sources and social media can be lousy sources of reliable medical information, they can be helpful places to share your experiences with other HIV-positive people in an anonymous setting.

You should also inform your healthcare providers, including doctors, dentists, counselors, and therapists. They need to know your HIV status to be able to take care of your properly. If you have a provider you don't feel you can tell, then it's probably time to change providers.

You *don't* have to tell your boss, your coworkers, your plumber, or the guy sitting next to you on the bus.

5. Should I keep working?

Yes! Most people with HIV continue to work. You've got a long life ahead of you, and you're going to need the money and insurance, not to mention the opportunity to remain productive and to maintain a sense of purpose.

If you're sick now, with a low CD4 cell count or a complication from HIV, it may be necessary to take time out of work and focus on your health. You should make getting healthy your top priority. But your disability should be temporary—you'll get a lot better once you start treatment. In rare situations, HIV can sometimes lead to permanent disability despite treatment, especially in people with advanced disease or in those who develop severe complications with long-lasting consequences. If you feel you can't work, talk to your provider, a social worker, or a case manager. You may qualify for temporary or permanent disability payments either through your employer, private disability insurance, **Social Security Disability Insurance (SSDI)**, or **Supplemental Security Income (SSI)**. If you intend to keep working but expect frequent absences due to illness or medical visits or health problems, consider filing for benefits under the **Family Medical Leave Act (FMLA)**, which will protect your job during those absences. Information on FMLA is available online or through your employer's human resources department.

If you were once sick from HIV and are now doing well, you may be receiving permanent disability payments because of complications that happened years ago. You

Social Security Disability Insurance (SSDI)

A monthly Social Security benefit for disabled people who have worked in the past and have paid a minimum amount for Social Security taxes.

Supplemental Security Income (SSI)

A federal cash assistance program designed to help the aged, blind, and disabled who have little or no income to pay for basic necessities.

Family Medical Leave Act (FMLA)

A federal law that allows people to take time off work without fear of termination or loss of benefits to deal with their own serious or chronic medical problems or those of their family members. People who need this protection must file paperwork with their employers in advance.

have two options—you can continue to receive disability payments or give them up and return to work.

This can be a tough decision. It's hard to go back to work after years of not working, to explain long gaps in your employment history to a prospective employer, to give up a steady income, and to give up other benefits that often come with being on disability, including Medicare. On the other hand, disability isn't guaranteed for life. Applications have to be renewed frequently, and unless your medical records indicate that you're *currently* disabled, the checks could stop. Your doctor may not feel comfortable putting down on a form that you are disabled if you've regained your health.

If you feel you're able to return to work after a period of time on disability, there are federal and state transition programs that offer return-to-work programs and benefits. If you're wrestling with this decision, talk it over with your provider, social worker, or case manager.

6. But I don't know! Should I get tested?

This is the easiest question in the book—YES! HIV testing is recommended for *all* adults and adolescents, which means that *everyone* should know his or her HIV status. (You could disregard this recommendation if you've never had sex or shared needles.)

In general we'd be a lot better off if we stopped worrying about "risk factors" and just tested everybody—that's what the Centers for Disease Control (CDC) recommended in 2006. We have a simple, cheap, highly accurate test for a disease that's spread from person to person, is highly treatable, and is fatal if untreated. It's tragic that about 1 in 6 HIV-positive Americans don't

---

Routine HIV testing is now recommended for all adults and adolescents, which means that almost everyone should know his or her HIV status.

Fourth-generation HIV tests

HIV tests that detect both antigen and antibody, allowing them to detect HIV sooner after infection than other antibody tests.

Sexually transmitted infections (STIs)

Infection transmitted from person to person through sexual activity. Also called sexually transmitted diseases (STDs).

Hepatitis B

An acute or chronic viral infection of the liver caused by the hepatitis B virus (HBV).

know they have HIV, leading to unnecessary death, illness, and transmission of the virus to others.

People often get tested because they're afraid they might have been infected from a specific event, and they often obsess about the "window period": the time between infection and a positive test result. With the older HIV tests, most people had positive results within 2 to 8 weeks, and between 97% and 99.7% were positive within 3 months. The newer tests (**fourth-generation HIV tests**), which measure both HIV antigen *and* antibody, detect HIV earlier. Ninety-five percent of recently infected people will have positive results within 1 to 8 weeks (Question 15).

If you're sexually active—and especially if you're having unprotected sex—it makes more sense to get tested every 6 to 12 months rather than try to time the test based on the exposure, which can drive you (and your medical provider) crazy.

So everyone should be tested at least once: that's easy. There are certain conditions for which testing is *especially* recommended—people who've had a **sexually transmitted infection (STI)**, **hepatitis B**, **hepatitis C, tuberculosis (TB)**, **shingles (herpes zoster),** or problems that could be caused by HIV, such as weight loss or chronic diarrhea. HIV testing should be performed in anyone with lymphoma or unexplained **thrombocytopenia** (low platelet count), anemia (low red blood cell count), or **leukopenia** (low white blood cell count). All pregnant women should be tested because treatment prevents transmission to their infants.

Hepatitis C

An acute or chronic viral infection of the liver caused by the hepatitis C virus (HCV).

Tuberculosis (TB)

A bacterial disease caused by *Mycobacterium tuberculosis.* TB most often causes lung disease but can affect any part of the body.

Shingles (or herpes zoster)

A painful, blistering rash, usually occurring in a linear band on one side of the body, caused by reactivation of the chickenpox virus (varicella-zoster virus, VZV).

Thrombocytopenia

A disorder in which there is an abnormally low number of platelets in the blood.

Leukopenia

A decrease in the number of white blood cells found in the blood.

PART TWO

The Basics

What's the difference between HIV and AIDS?

How is HIV spread?

How can HIV be prevented? What is PrEP?

More . . .

HIV

Human immunode-
ficiency virus, the
virus that causes HIV
infection and AIDS.

AIDS

Acquired immunode-
ficiency syndrome, a
more advanced stage
of HIV defined by
having a CD4 count
below 200 or one of a
list of AIDS-indicator
conditions (see
Table 1).

Life cycle

In HIV infection, the
stages that the virus
goes through, start-
ing with its entry into
human cells and end-
ing with its replica-
tion and the release
of new virus particles
into the blood.

7. What is HIV?

HIV stands for "**h**uman **i**mmunodeficiency **v**irus," the virus that causes **AIDS** (**a**cquired **i**mmunodeficiency **s**yndrome). The difference between HIV and AIDS is discussed in Question 10. HIV is passed from person to person through sexual contact, blood exposure, child-birth, and breastfeeding (Question 12).

It's time to take a brief detour into the basic science of the **life cycle** of HIV—I promise to make it short. For even more details, see Question 29, and refer to **Figure 1** because a picture will make this easier to understand.

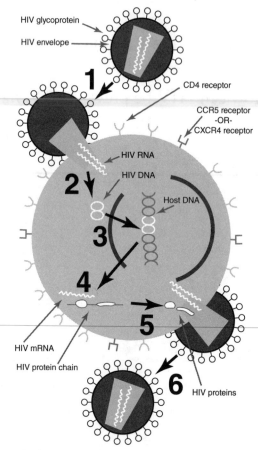

Figure 1 The HIV life cycle.

HIV is a **retrovirus**, a virus that contains **enzymes** (proteins) that can turn **RNA**, its genetic material, into DNA. It's called a retrovirus because this is the reverse of most viruses, in which DNA is converted through the process of **transcription** into RNA. After infection, HIV RNA gets turned into DNA by the **reverse transcriptase** (RT) enzyme, an enzyme that comes with the virus. That viral DNA is then inserted into

The HIV Life Cycle

1. **Entry**: CD4 attachment, co-receptor finding, and fusion. HIV begins its life cycle when it attaches to a CD4 receptor and then binds to one of two co-receptors (CCR5 or CXCR4) on the surface of the CD4 cell. The envelope (coating) of the virus then fuses with the CD4 cell. After fusion, the virus inserts its RNA (genetic material) into the host cell.

2. **Reverse transcription**: An HIV enzyme (protein) called "reverse transcriptase" converts the RNA of the virus into HIV DNA.

3. **Integration**: The newly formed HIV DNA enters the nucleus of the CD4 cell, where an HIV enzyme called "integrase" inserts it into the human DNA of the CD4 cell. The DNA of the virus can remain hidden for many years in resting CD4 cells, or it can be used to create new virus in activated CD4 cells.

4. **Transcription and translation**: In an activated CD4 cell, the HIV DNA is transcribed into RNA, which is then translated into HIV proteins.

5. **Assembly**: An HIV enzyme called "protease" cuts long chains of HIV proteins into smaller individual proteins. New virus particles are assembled from the smaller HIV proteins and copies of HIV RNA.

6. **Budding**: The newly assembled virus buds push out from the CD4 cell. The new copies of HIV are now free to infect other cells.

Adapted with permission from AIDSinfo, a DHHS information service managed by NIH.

Retrovirus

A virus that contains RNA and that can turn RNA into DNA through reverse transcription using viral enzymes. HIV is a retrovirus.

Enzymes

Proteins that carry out a biological function. Examples of enzymes carried by HIV include reverse transcriptase, integrase, and protease. Each plays a role in allowing the virus to reproduce, and each is a target for antiretroviral therapy.

RNA

Ribonucleic acid, the genetic material of the HIV virus. Viral RNA gets turned into DNA by reverse transcriptase, and the viral DNA then gets inserted into the DNA of human cells. DNA is later transcribed back into RNA, which in turn gets translated into the proteins that are used to make new virus particles.

Transcription

The process of turning DNA into RNA.

Reverse transcriptase (RT)

An enzyme contained within the HIV virus that turns viral RNA into DNA so it can be inserted into the DNA of human cells. A reverse transcriptase inhibitor blocks this process.

Reservoir

Long-lived human cells that can be infected by HIV, allowing it to persist (remain latent) for the lifetime of the individual, even if they are on antiretroviral therapy with an "undetectable" viral load. Resting CD4 cells are the best known example, but there are other reservoirs in the human body.

Resting CD4 cells

CD4 cells that live a long time and can harbor HIV DNA, which can't be affected by ART because the cell is not replicating, and thus are an important reservoir of latent HIV.

Pandemic

A global epidemic.

the DNA of human cells. The viral DNA can then be translated into viral proteins, which form new viruses that go on to infect new cells. Unfortunately, the virus can also remain latent in long-lived cells (**reservoirs**) such as **resting CD4 cells** or brain cells, where it can't be reached by antiretroviral drugs. HIV's ability to remain latent is what allows it to persist for life, even with effective treatment. It's what has kept us from finding a cure so far (Question 14).

When it's not treated, HIV causes progressive damage to the immune system and is almost always fatal. It is the world's most serious **pandemic** (a global **epidemic**), and there are no immediate prospects for either a cure or a preventive **vaccine** (**vaccination**). Fortunately, treatment today is highly effective, and deaths from HIV disease are now mostly preventable in countries where therapy is available and affordable. And death from HIV is *completely* preventable if treatment is started before the immune system is weakened! I'm very confident telling people with HIV that happy information.

8. Where did HIV come from?

Research now shows that **HIV-1**,* the most common type of HIV worldwide, first infected humans in sub-Saharan Africa at some point in the first half of the 20th century. It was transmitted from chimpanzees when people came into contact with their blood through hunting or butchering. HIV probably remained confined to Africa for many decades, in part

---

*HIV-2 is a related but less common virus found almost exclusively in West Africa. Standard blood tests will detect both viruses.

because travel within and from Africa was uncommon then. We have definite proof of human HIV in Africa dating back to 1959.

The virus eventually spread beyond Africa, probably entering the United States in the mid- to late 1970s. Unusual cases of rare infections and cancers began to be seen in gay and bisexual men between 1979 and 1981, and the AIDS epidemic is said to have begun when these reports first appeared in medical journals in 1981, making it clear that there was an emerging epidemic. In hindsight, many doctors recall seeing people with HIV disease before 1981, especially in cities with large numbers of cases such as New York City, Los Angeles, and San Francisco. HIV was discovered in 1983, leading to an accurate blood test and eventually to treatment.

The disease was originally reported in gay and bisexual men, but the "risk groups" were later expanded to include injection drug users and people with hemophilia. It eventually became clear that "risk behaviors" were more important than "risk groups." People could be infected through unprotected sex, exposure to infected blood, or childbirth or breastfeeding. It's estimated that more than 36 million children and adults were infected with HIV worldwide as of 2017.

9. How does HIV make you sick?

HIV causes illness mainly by damaging the immune system, which protects us from getting infections and cancers. HIV's most important target is the **CD4 cell** (also known as the **CD4 lymphocyte** or **T-helper cell**).

Epidemic

The appearance of new cases of disease (especially an infectious disease) in a human population at a higher rate than would be expected.

Vaccine (vaccination)

A substance that is given, usually by injection but sometimes by mouth or by nasal spray, to stimulate the immune system to make antibodies against a bacterial or viral pathogen.

HIV-1

The most common form of HIV worldwide.

CD4 cell (or CD4 lymphocyte or T-helper cell)

A type of lymphocyte (a type of white blood cell) that can be infected by HIV. CD4 cells fight certain infections and cancers. The number of CD4 cells (CD4 count) declines with untreated HIV, which leads to weakening of the immune system, also called immunosuppression.

White blood cell (WBC)

A type of blood cell that helps fight infection. CD4 cells are a type of lymphocyte, which is a type of white blood cell.

The CD4 cell is a type of **white blood cell** (**WBC**) responsible for controlling or preventing infection with many common viruses, bacteria, fungi, and parasites, as well as some cancers. HIV destruction of CD4 cells. Over time, the number of CD4 cells (the CD4 count) declines. Although it may take many years, the CD4 count eventually becomes so low that there aren't enough cells to fight certain infections or cancers, which allows complications to occur. The speed at which the CD4 count falls varies from person to person and depends on a number of factors, including genetic characteristics, characteristics of the viral strain, and the amount of virus in the blood (viral load).

Immune activation

A general stimulation of the immune system that can be caused by a variety of infections, including HIV infection. In the case of HIV, it is thought to cause the decline in CD4 count that occurs with time.

There are several reasons why the CD4 cell count drops. The virus directly infects some CD4 cells, which leads to their decline. More important, HIV causes a chronic **immune activation** (stimulation of the immune system), which may be responsible for the reduction in the number of CD4 cells. Chronic inflammation may also increase the long-term risk of certain medical conditions, such as coronary heart disease, cancers, or other conditions that become more common as we age (Questions 47 and 61).

In addition to damaging the immune system, HIV can directly affect many of the body's organs, such as the nervous system (Question 73) and the kidneys (Question 49). It can also cause weight loss, night sweats, and diarrhea (Question 11). When deaths due to AIDS were common, it was often said that people didn't die of HIV itself but of one of its complications, such as a cancer or infection. While that was technically true in most cases, HIV was still the underlying problem that led to death from AIDS.

10. What's the difference between HIV and AIDS?

The term *AIDS* was coined in 1982. It stands for "acquired immunodeficiency syndrome." It's "acquired" to show that it was not something a person was born with (those are "congenital"). **Immunodeficiency** (or **immunosuppression**) means the immune system is weakened. It's a **syndrome** because in the years before HIV was discovered and identified as the cause of AIDS, we recognized a collection of symptoms and complications, including infections and cancers that occurred in people who had common risk factors.

Importantly, back when the term AIDS was first used, HIV hadn't been discovered yet. Someone was said to have AIDS if he or she developed one of a long list of complications, either **opportunistic infections (OIs)** or cancers, that don't occur in people with healthy immune systems (Question 53). After HIV was discovered and a blood test became available, the definition of AIDS changed so that having a positive HIV test (in addition to the complication) was required to say someone had AIDS. In 1993, the **Centers for Disease Control and Prevention (CDC)** expanded the definition of AIDS to include people with HIV whose CD4 counts were less than 200, even if they didn't have complications. The current **AIDS case definition** is shown in **Table 1**.

So the bottom line of this sometimes confusing distinction is that everyone who has AIDS has HIV, but not everyone with HIV has AIDS. Some have advocated no longer using the term AIDS, as it is more associated with illness and stigma than HIV. However, as a description of people who are (or were) once sick with complications from HIV, it still serves some purpose.

Immunodeficiency (or immunosuppression)

A state in which the immune system is damaged or impaired, either from birth (congenital immunodeficiency) or acquired, as in HIV.

Syndrome

A collection of signs or symptoms that frequently occur together but that may or may not be caused by a single disease. AIDS was referred to as a syndrome before its cause, HIV, had been discovered.

Opportunistic infection (OI)

An infection that takes advantage of immunodeficiency. These infections usually don't occur in people with normal immune systems.

Centers for Disease Control and Prevention (CDC)

A branch of the federal government, within the U.S. Department of Health and Human Services (HHS), that is charged with tracking, preventing, and controlling health problems in the United States, including infectious diseases such as HIV.

AIDS case definition

The criteria used by the CDC to classify someone as having AIDS.

Table 1 AIDS-Indicator Conditions (CDC AIDS Case Definition, 1993)

Candidal esophagitis [65]* (or candidiasis of the respiratory tract, which is rare)

Cervical cancer, invasive [61, 81]

Coccidioidomycosis involving an organ other than the lungs [57]

Cryptococcosis involving an organ other than the lungs [57]

Cryptosporidiosis with diarrhea for at least 1 month [66, 90]

CMV disease involving an organ other than the liver, spleen, or lymph nodes [58]

Herpes simplex with ulcers lasting more than 1 month [89] or with esophagitis [65] or infection of the respiratory tract (rare)

Histoplasmosis involving an organ other than the lungs [57]

HIV-associated dementia [73]

Isosporiasis (a parasitic disease that is uncommon in the United States) with diarrhea for at least 1 month [66]

Kaposi's sarcoma [61]

Lymphoma [61]

Mycobacterium avium complex (MAC) [55], *Mycobacterium kansasii*, or other mycobacterial infection involving organs other than the lungs

Tuberculosis [59]

Pneumocystis pneumonia (PCP) [54]

Pneumonia, bacterial: two or more episodes in 1 year [67]

Progressive multifocal leukoencephalopathy (PML) [72]

Salmonella with bloodstream infection, recurrent [66]

Toxoplasmosis [56]

Wasting syndrome (greater than 10% weight loss plus chronic diarrhea, weakness, or fever lasting more than 30 days) [69]

*Numbers in brackets refer to questions in which the topics are discussed.
Reproduced from the Centers for Disease Control and Prevention.

One term definitely to avoid is "full-blown AIDS." Another one is "end-stage AIDS". These are outdated, unnecessarily scary, and not helpful. If you're HIV positive, the disease you have is HIV. (You'll sometimes see it referred to as **HIV disease**. Some have objected to using the word "infection", so I typically just say "HIV".) AIDS just refers to a more advanced stage of that disease. Treatment can prevent HIV from turning

HIV disease

The name for the disease caused by HIV. AIDS is a late, or more advanced, stage of HIV.

into AIDS, and it can restore the health of people with AIDS. In the eyes of the people who keep track of the epidemic, once you have AIDS, you'll always have AIDS. But what should matter to you and your provider is how you're doing *now*.

11. What are the stages of HIV?

The first stage of HIV, occurring a few weeks after a person gets the virus, is called **acute HIV**, or **primary HIV**. The symptoms people experience during this illness are called the **acute retroviral syndrome (ARS)** (Question 16). During acute HIV, some HIV tests, especially antibody tests, are negative, but the amount of virus in the blood (measured by the viral load) is extremely high, making it easy to transmit HIV to others. Newer tests screen for both HIV antibody and **antigen** (actual parts of HIV), so the test is much more accurate than it used to be during acute HIV. These newer tests are sometimes called the "4th-Generation" HIV screening tests to distinguish them from the earlier tests that only checked for antibody.

The symptoms of acute HIV resolve on their own and acute HIV is followed by a latent stage, usually called **asymptomatic HIV**. People generally feel fine during that stage, although their **lymph nodes** may be enlarged (**lymphadenopathy**), and some common conditions can occur more often or be more severe, including vaginal yeast infections, herpes, or shingles.

Some people develop symptoms of HIV before actually developing AIDS. This stage is referred to as **symptomatic HIV** (formerly **AIDS-related complex**, or **ARC**). Symptoms include weight loss, oral **thrush** (a **yeast** infection in the mouth), diarrhea, night sweats, and fatigue.

THE BASICS

Acute (or primary) HIV

The stage of HIV infection that occurs shortly after infection. At this stage, the viral load is very high. People often have symptoms during this stage.

Acute retroviral syndrome (ARS)

A collection of symptoms, such as fever, rash, sore throat, and swollen lymph nodes, that many people experience during acute infection, shortly after they're infected.

Asymptomatic HIV

An early stage of HIV infection in which infected people have a positive test but no symptoms.

Lymph nodes

Structures of the human body that are part of the immune system. You might feel them in the neck, under the arms, or in the groin.

Lymphadenopathy

Swollen or enlarged lymph nodes ("glands").

A person is considered to have AIDS if the CD4 count falls below 200 (whether or not you have symptoms) or when an **AIDS-indicator condition** (or **AIDS-defining condition**) has been diagnosed (see Table 1). Most people reach a CD4 count of 200 before developing complications, so a low CD4 count is the most common reason for an AIDS diagnosis. As the CD4 count declines further, the list of possible complications grows. We sometimes refer to someone with a CD4 count below 50 as having **advanced HIV disease**. Before we had effective HIV treatment, most of the deaths related to HIV occurred when the CD4 count was below 50.

If it's not diagnosed and treated, HIV almost always progresses from early stages to late stages, eventually resulting in illness and death. Treatment can move you from a late stage back to an early stage. Fortunately, HIV is treatable at *any* stage, and treatment can restore health even for people with advanced HIV.

12. How is HIV spread?

There are only a few ways in which HIV can be spread:

- *Sexual transmission.* For HIV to be spread through sex, the semen, vaginal fluids, or blood of an infected person must enter the body of an uninfected person. This usually happens through vaginal or anal intercourse. The risk is greatest if the "insertive" partner (the "top") is positive, but the top can be infected by the receptive partner (the "bottom"), too. Transmission through oral sex is much less common, but it can happen. (For a more detailed discussion of the risks of specific sexual activities and reducing sexual risk, see Questions 13 and 86.)

- *Blood exposure.* HIV can be transmitted through transfusion, though the risk is virtually nonexistent in places where the blood supply is tested. Far more commonly, it's transmitted through injection drug use, when negative users share needles or syringes ("works") with positive users. Healthcare workers have been infected when they've been stuck with needles containing infected blood or when their eyes, nose, or open cuts have been splashed with blood or body fluids from an HIV-positive patient.
- *Childbirth and breastfeeding.* HIV-infected women can pass HIV to their infants during childbirth (usually at the time of labor or shortly before) or by breastfeeding (Question 76). Infants aren't infected at the time of conception, so an HIV-positive man can only infect the infant indirectly, by infecting the mother.

HIV isn't spread through contact with saliva, urine, sweat, or feces. Contrary to popular belief, it is *not* transmitted by mosquitoes, exposure of body fluids to intact skin, holding hands, kissing, hugging, sharing drinking glasses or eating utensils, mutual masturbation, or having naughty thoughts!

13. How can HIV be prevented? What is PrEP?

HIV is a *completely* preventable disease. Here's what you need to know about prevention, organized by the type of transmission:

- *Sexual transmission, HIV-negative people.* It doesn't get any safer than abstinence. But while this approach has its supporters, it's not acceptable to everyone, and even among the most vocal proponents

AIDS-indicator condition (or AIDS-defining condition)

One of a list of conditions, including opportunistic infections and malignancies, that is used by the CDC to determine who has AIDS (see Table 1).

Advanced HIV disease

The most advanced stage of HIV, usually in people with CD4 counts below 50.

of abstinence, "sex happens." The next best alternatives are to (1) limit the number of sexual partners; (2) engage in sexual activities other than anal or vaginal intercourse; (3) avoid getting semen, pre-seminal fluid ("pre-cum"), and vaginal fluids in your mouth or eyes; (4) use condoms when you *do* have intercourse; and (5) use **pre-exposure prophylaxis (PrEP)**, especially if you're not always using condoms. For more details on safer sexual practices, see Question 86. HIV-negative people should play it safe regardless of what they're told about their partners' status. Partners don't always know or reveal their current status, or their status may change.

Pre-exposure prophylaxis (PrEP)

A form of HIV prevention in which antiretroviral medications are taken by HIV-negative individuals to prevent infection.

Research now has conclusively shown that if people are taking ART faithfully, and the viral load is suppressed by treatment, that they cannot pass the virus on to others sexually. So if you're in a couple where your partner has HIV and you don't, the most effective way to avoid getting HIV is for your partner to be on ART!

If you're HIV negative and you're not always using condoms during sex, PrEP is a highly effective way to prevent HIV. This currently involves taking Truvada or Descovy (pills containing two antiretroviral agents, tenofovir and emtricitabine) once daily to prevent transmission. It won't prevent other sexually transmitted infections, but it will probably keep you from getting HIV, provided you take it regularly. New forms of PrEP are being studied, including long-acting injections. Intermittent or "on-demand" PrEP (taken only around the time of sexual activity) is also being studied, and there were some promising results from a French study. The way they took PrEP in this study was to take 2 pills the day before sex and 1 pill the next two days.

This method of taking PrEP should be considered an alternative to daily PrEP in people who can't remember to take it daily.

- *Sexual transmission, HIV-positive people.* If you're HIV positive, it's your responsibility to never infect anyone else (regardless of the behavior or preferences of your partners). Condoms are effective when used regularly and correctly, but they don't work when left unopened in the nightstand drawer. Even more important than condoms is being on effective ART with an undetectable viral load (Questions 28 and 86), which is the most important way for positive people to avoid infecting others. As noted above, it's now been shown in multiple studies that people who have HIV can't transmit the virus to others sexually if they're taking ART. This message of "Undetectable = Untransmissable," or "U = U" has become a big motivation for people to take ART!

- *Drug use.* The best way to prevent infection from drug use is to get treatment to help you stop using. But if you're going to use drugs, don't share needles and syringes. That can be easier said than done, especially in places that don't have needle exchange programs. If you do share syringes and needles, decontaminate them with bleach after every use. PrEP has also been shown to protect drug users against HIV.

- *Transmission to infants.* All pregnant women should be tested for HIV. Provided it's started early enough in pregnancy, treatment during pregnancy is nearly 100% effective at preventing transmission to the baby (Question 76). HIV-positive women should not breastfeed their babies.

Don't spend time worrying about obscure ways of getting infected. The simple fact is that if all HIV-positive people were diagnosed and on effective ART, the HIV epidemic would come to an end. Short of that, we can achieve almost the same outcome with broader use of condoms, PrEP, and needle exchange.

14. Why isn't there a cure?

Given how long the disease has been around, it may seem strange that we haven't found a cure for HIV yet. Conspiracy theorists argue that a cure exists but is being suppressed by profit-motivated drug companies or by evil governments trying to cull their populations of "less desirable" elements. I'll leave that discussion for later (Question 98) and will talk about science here.

Some viruses get better on their own (the common cold), some remain dormant in your body forever (herpes), some are preventable with vaccination (measles), and some scary ones can be deadly very quickly (rabies, ebola)! The fact that HIV hides out by inserting its DNA into long-lived human cells makes it a difficult problem to tackle, but fortunately it doesn't fall into this last frightening group!

To put HIV into perspective, many diseases that we suffer from in the developed world are *also* chronic, incurable—but treatable diseases. Think of diabetes, coronary artery disease, congestive heart failure, and arthritis. None of them is curable, but all of them are manageable. Amazingly, they tend to be harder to manage than HIV.

Unlike the early years of HIV, there now is a lot of research looking into curing HIV. You may have heard about Timothy Ray Brown, "the Berlin patient," an HIV-positive man with leukemia who has been cured of HIV after getting a bone marrow transplant using marrow from a donor who was genetically immune to HIV because of the **delta 32 mutation**, the absence of CCR5 coreceptors on the surface of the CD4 cell (Question 27). Now a second person looks like he has been cured with a similar procedure. Unfortunately, bone marrow transplants are expensive, risky procedures, done only for people who would otherwise die of their underlying condition (usually cancer) if they didn't get them.

Also, people who get them require lifelong immunosuppression to prevent rejection. But these two cases tell us that cure is possible and may point us to safer ways to achieve this goal.

There are a number of cure strategies that are under study. **Latency-reversing agents** are drugs that activate or "wake up" infected resting CD4 cells. They're being studied in a **shock and kill** approach, where you attack the replicating virus with antiretroviral drugs after activating it with latency-reversing agents.

Another strategy, genetically modifying CD4 cells to make them uninfectable—like the cells that the two cure cases received in their bone marrow transplants—preventing HIV from infecting new cells. Immune-based therapies and therapeutic vaccines could help the immune system fight HIV on its own.

A cure could be "sterilizing" (the virus is completely eradicated) or "functional" (HIV is still present, but the immune system keeps it under control without ART). Cure and eradication research is now a high priority

Delta 32 mutation

A genetic condition resulting in the absence of CCR5 coreceptor on the CD4 cell. Individuals who are heterozygous for this deletion (the mutation is present in only one copy of the gene) can be infected by HIV but progress more slowly. Those who are homozygous (the mutation is present in both copies of the gene) cannot be infected by R5 virus, the most common form of circulating HIV.

Latency-reversing agents

Drugs being studied in experimental cure strategies that activate HIV-infected resting CD4 cells in order to eliminate the latent reservoir.

Shock and kill

An experimental cure strategy in which HIV-infected resting CD4 cells are first activated by latency-reversing agents, allowing the virus to be treated with antiretroviral therapy.

at the National Institutes of Health (NIH) and world-wide. Provided we continue to generously fund scientific research, the search for a cure will continue to be the focus of some of our best scientists.

In about 15 years, we saw HIV go from being an almost universally fatal, untreatable illness to a manageable, chronic disease.

In the meantime, it would be a mistake to look at cure as the only measure of success. In just 15 years, we saw HIV go from being an almost universally fatal, untreatable illness to a manageable, chronic disease—and treatment became easier and better in the years that followed. A cure will be a scientific breakthrough of unprecedented proportions; until then, we'll have to be content with triumphant, unparalleled success.

PART THREE

Diagnosis

How is HIV diagnosed?

How do I know if I've been recently infected?

What if all of my tests are negative, but I'm sure that I have HIV?

More . . .

15. How is HIV diagnosed?

Tests to diagnose HIV are *highly* accurate. The traditional strategy using the older, third-generation antibody tests was to screen first with an **enzyme-linked immunoassay** (**ELISA** or **EIA**). Now, a **4th-Generation Screening Test** is more commonly done first. This checks for both **antibody** (a protein your body makes in response to the virus) *and* **antigen** (an actual part of the virus). This new 4th-Generation test has the advantage of turning positive much sooner after getting HIV than the antibody-only test it replaced. Blood tests that measure antibodies are sometimes called **serologies**.

If the screening test is positive, the lab automatically runs a confirmatory test called a **differentiation assay**, which is an antibody test that detects whether you have HIV-1, or HIV-2, or neither. A false-positive test in both the screening test and the differentiation assay are extremely rare. When they happen, it's usually due to a mistake made by someone doing the lab test—a mislabeled tube or the wrong name on the lab report. The differentiation assay replaced a test called the Western blot, which only checked for antibodies to HIV-1.

An **indeterminate HIV test** means the screening test is positive and the differentiation assay is negative. This can occur for one of two reasons. First, you might have been recently infected and are in the process of **seroconversion**—in this case, the screening test picked up the antigen (actually part of the virus), but your body hasn't had a chance yet to develop antibody (development of a positive differentiation assay). The second possibility is that the screening test might have been a false-positive.

Enzyme-linked immunoassay (ELISA or EIA)
A test that detects and measures antibodies in your blood.

4th-generation screening test
The initial test done to diagnose HIV, detecting both antibodies and HIV antigen. Positive tests must be confirmed with a differentiation assay.

Antibody
Proteins used by the immune system to fight infection.

Antigen
Proteins from organisms, such as bacteria or viruses, that stimulate an immune response.

Serologies
Blood tests that measure antibodies to look for evidence of a disease.

Differentiation assay
A confirmatory antibody test that detects whether HIV antibody is present and whether the antibody is to HIV-1 or to HIV-2.

How does someone tell if you are seroconverting versus just have a false-positive screening test? Fortunately, this can be accomplished very accurately by sending an HIV viral load. If the HIV viral load is positive, it will usually be very high, indicating that a person has recently acquired HIV. If it's negative, or **undetectable**, then the screening test was a false-positive—and nothing to worry about! It can be scary to have a false-positive screening test, but the good news is that it has no bearing on your health.

Rapid tests give results within a few minutes and are available in many clinics, especially those that test for other sexually transmitted infections. These are great for getting results even before you leave the clinic. An important limitation to these tests is that they are not quite as accurate as lab-based tests, so the results need to be confirmed with a lab-based test if they are positive. For **home testing**, *OraQuick* (www.oraquick.com) uses an oral swab and also provides immediate results. Follow the instructions to the letter because *OraQuick* has been somewhat less accurate when performed by laypeople than by laboratory or medical personnel. If you have any doubt about the test result, it makes sense to have a regular lab-based test.

16. How do I know if I've been recently infected?

Most people feel sick within a few weeks of getting HIV. This is called "acute (or primary) infection," and the symptoms (illness) that occur may be called the "acute retroviral syndrome" (ARS), or acute HIV (Question 11). The illness may be mild and brief, or it may be severe enough to require hospitalization. In most cases,

Indeterminate HIV test

This occurs when the screening test is positive, but the differentiation assay is negative. This can occur during the process of seroconversion (recently acquired HIV) or it can be found in people without HIV, usually for unclear reasons.

Seroconversion

The process of developing an antibody to an infectious agent. In the case of HIV, it occurs within 2-4 weeks after acute infection.

Undetectable

A term used to describe a viral load that is too low to be measured by a viral load test. An undetectable viral load is below 20, 30, or 40 with the most commonly used tests.

Rapid tests

HIV tests that provide an answer within a few minutes, using either blood or saliva.

Home tests

An HIV blood or oral test that can be performed at home.

Bell's palsy

A paralysis of one side of the face that can be caused by a variety of infections, including acute HIV.

Aseptic meningitis

Meningitis that is not caused by a bacterium that can be grown in culture. Can be caused by viruses (including HIV during acute HIV) or drugs.

Guillain-Barré syndrome

Progressive muscle paralysis starting in the legs and moving upward, sometimes seen during acute HIV.

Myopathy

An inflammation of muscles causing muscle pain and weakness, sometimes seen with acute retroviral syndrome, high-dose zidovudine, or statin drugs used to lower cholesterol.

Window period

The period between infection and formation of antibodies leading to a positive HIV test (serology).

the symptoms are similar to those of mononucleosis. They can include any of fever, rash, muscle aches, fatigue, sore throat, swollen lymph nodes, diarrhea, and weight loss. Less often, people can develop neurologic symptoms, such as **Bell's palsy** (paralysis of one side of the face), **aseptic meningitis**, **Guillain-Barré syndrome** (paralysis that starts in the legs and moves up the body), or **myopathy** (muscle pain and weakness). Sometimes, people with ARS become seriously immunosuppressed and develop opportunistic infections that normally occur only in people with longstanding HIV disease, but this happens very rarely.

During acute HIV, the fourth-generation screening test is usually positive since it detects HIV antigen as well as antibody. However, the differentiation assay is often negative unless a person has been sick already for a couple of weeks. This period between acquiring an infection and the antibody turning positive is sometimes called the **window period**, which in HIV is typically 2 to 4 weeks. Because of the window period, your providers should order an HIV viral load if they suspect acute HIV. If it is truly acute HIV, the viral load will be high (hundreds of thousands or even millions). By contrast, if the viral load is undetectable, HIV is *not* the cause of these symptoms. Your doctor should consider other causes of your illness.

Unfortunately, the diagnosis of acute HIV is too often missed. The symptoms are nonspecific (common to other viral conditions), and many healthcare providers either don't think about HIV or don't know how to diagnose it. You can help the clinicians who are evaluating you by sharing with them that you are concerned you might have recently contracted HIV. This will increase the chances they will order the correct tests.

It's important to diagnose HIV at this stage for several reasons. First, people with acute HIV have extremely high levels of HIV in their blood, semen, and vaginal fluids, making it easy for them to spread HIV to others if they don't know they're positive. Second, it's possible to have acquired a drug-resistant HIV (virus that isn't suppressed by one or more drugs; see Question 38). The best time to test for transmitted resistance is during acute HIV (Question 24). Finally, there is benefit to starting treatment during acute HIV rather than waiting. Starting treatment *very* early preserves your CD4 cells at their highest level. Plus, treatment at this early stage may reduce the size of the latent reservoir, and it's thought that such people will be the best candidates for a cure, when, not if, a cure becomes available!

17. What if all of my tests are negative, but I'm sure that I have HIV?

The good news is that HIV is *not* hard to diagnose. We're fortunate that testing for HIV is among the most accurate testing strategies in all of medicine! A negative HIV test after the appropriate window period for that test means you don't have HIV. You don't need a CD4 count, a DNA test, or a viral culture. You don't need to see a specialist. You don't need to think about rare subtypes or whether medications you take are causing false-negative tests results.

What you *may* need is a psychiatrist or a psychotherapist. Irrational obsession with disease can be a sign of depression, obsessive-compulsive disorder, or hypochondriasis. Depression and anxiety can cause many of the symptoms that lead people to think they have HIV. People may also obsess about HIV because it's easier than dealing with more difficult issues like guilt or anxiety about sexuality or infidelity.

HIV is not hard to diagnose.

PART FOUR

Medical Care

How do I find the right medical care?

What are my provider's responsibilities,
and what are mine?

How will I pay for medical care?

More . . .

18. How do I find the right medical care?

Choosing a medical provider is one of the most important decisions you make about your health, so make it carefully. (There are some people who don't like the word "provider," thinking it's too technical sounding. But it intends to cover doctors, nurses, physician assistants, social workers, pharmacists, and other members of a team who could be taking care of you. Sometimes I'll use the term "clinician," which means the same thing.) Treating HIV can be complex; it's not something that should be attempted by providers without experience and training. Studies have shown that people treated by HIV experts stay healthier and live longer than those managed by non-experts. Mistakes made by inexperienced clinicians early in the course of therapy can lead to drug resistance that never goes away. If your doctor says they haven't managed many people with HIV, find another doctor!

I use the term "expert" because there's technically no such thing as an "HIV specialist." A specialist is someone who has passed a specialty board exam, and there is no widely accepted exam for HIV. An HIV expert is a clinician with lots of HIV experience who keeps up with the latest research and developments in the field. Some infectious disease specialists are HIV experts, but some aren't. There are general internists and family practitioners who *are* HIV experts, but most aren't. Experts don't have to be doctors: There are expert nurse practitioners and physician assistants and pharmacists and social workers, plus a large group of specialists who

People treated by HIV experts stay healthier and live longer than those managed by nonexperts.

have a special interest in HIV. I'm lucky to work with psychiatrists, obstetricians, dermatologists, and others who all want to care for people with HIV. Seek these people out if you need them—you want them to be a part of your care team!

Finding expert care can be tricky. If you have a primary medical provider, they may be able to refer you to someone. Ask a **case manager** or someone at an **AIDS service organization** for a recommendation. Talk to friends with HIV or support group members. Look for an expert in your area on the website for the American Academy of HIV Medicine (www.aahivm.org) or the HIV Medicine Association (www.hivma.org).

Having HIV doesn't mean you have to give up your long-term primary provider. Many will happily continue to see you even if they don't know much about HIV, and have your HIV treatment managed by an HIV expert as a consultant. They will continue to help you for non-HIV related issues. What matters is that your HIV care be directed by an expert and that the expert and your primary provider communicate with each other.

19. How do I deal with my healthcare provider?

The provider who treats you for HIV will be an important person in your life for a long time. This is someone you should like, trust, respect, and communicate easily with. As with any long-term relationship, your first may not be "The One." Don't be afraid to shop around

Case manager
A person who helps coordinate your medical care, provides referrals for needed services, and determines whether you qualify for any assistance or entitlement programs.

AIDS service organization (ASO)
An organization that provides services to people with HIV.

a little. Here are a few questions you should ask when you start a relationship with a new provider:

1. *Are you covered by my insurance plan?* This question is usually answered by the office staff or by someone from your insurance company before you ever see the provider (who may not know).

2. *How much experience do you have with HIV? How do you keep up with the latest advances in the field?* These may seem like awkward questions, but only someone who doesn't have what it takes will answer them defensively.

3. *Will you be my primary provider, or will you act as a consultant? Who should I contact about urgent medical problems?* The answer to the questions may be up to you, the provider, or your insurance company, but it's important to clarify them early on.

4. *How often will I see you? When do I get lab work drawn—before the visit or on the same day?* Getting your blood tests done a week or more before your visit allows us to review the result when you come in. On the other hand, some people don't want to come to the clinic or hospital twice, so they get the blood test done on the same day of the visit. In my view, both approaches are fine—whatever works best for you.

5. *How do I reach you between visits for questions, new problems, or emergencies?* Many providers now use secure web portals to communicate with patients; others have special phone-in hours; others use nurses, physician assistants, or nurse practitioners for first contact. Email can be used, but remember it is not secure—mistakes have been made where confidential medical information was sent to the wrong person. As a

result, I strongly suggest avoiding email as a way of communicating unless the security can be guaranteed. Find out who covers your provider for questions and emergencies when the provider is not on call or is on vacation.

6. *Where would I go if I needed to be hospitalized?*
You'd like to think that a great provider would be affiliated with a great hospital, but it doesn't always work that way. Fortunately, hospitalization is no longer inevitable, as it was when we didn't have good treatment for HIV, but it's still worth considering whether you'd be comfortable going to the hospital where your provider admits patients. Also, it's now common to be cared for by hospitalists when you're an inpatient rather than by your own doctor. Hospitalists are doctors who treat only hospitalized patients and then turn the care back to the primary care provider after discharge.

20. What are my provider's responsibilities, and what are mine?

Because your relationship with your provider should be a partnership, there are mutual responsibilities that both parties should be aware of.

Your Provider's Responsibilities

1. To treat you with respect and to pay attention to your concerns and opinions.
2. To ensure that urgent medical care is available to you at all times.
3. To keep you informed about your health status, your progress, and your prognosis in a language you can understand.

4. To tell you about your treatment options and to be willing to provide advice about which option he or she thinks is best.

5. To inform you of important side effects or long-term toxicities of medications and to help you weigh the risks and benefits of therapy (without overwhelming you with a long list of bad things that rarely happen).

Your Responsibilities

1. To treat the provider and staff with respect.

2. To provide a complete history, even if it means tracking down old medical records yourself. Better yet, keep your own records! See **Table 2** for a list of things you should keep track of.

3. To keep appointments or to cancel them with plenty of notice whenever possible.

4. To follow the course of treatment agreed on and to let the provider know about problems early so that treatment can be changed.

5. To be honest about what's going on in your life and with your treatment—even if it means disappointing your provider. We'd much rather know that you started smoking again (to use a common example) than have you hide this important medical history from us!

21. How will I pay for medical care?

Because this book is written from a U.S. perspective, the answer is complex. We have never really had a "health-care system" in this country; we've had multiple systems that depend on where you live, how old you are, if you're

Table 2 Information to Keep Track of and Share with New Providers

Dates

Date of HIV diagnosis

Approximate date of infection, if known (dates of exposure, previous negative tests, acute retroviral syndrome, etc.)

Dates of major complications

Test results (with dates)

CD4 counts

Viral loads

Resistance tests (genotypes and phenotypes)

Hepatitis A, B, and C serologies

Toxoplasma IgG antibody

Syphilis tests

Gonorrhea and chlamydia tests

Pap smears (cervical and/or anal)

Tests for latent TB infection (tuberculin skin test or interferon-gamma releasing assay)

Other tests, if applicable (HLA B*5701, tropism assay, etc.)

Vaccinations (with dates)

Tetanus (dT or Tdap)

Pneumococcal (*Pneumovax, Prevnar 13*)

Hepatitis A

Hepatitis B

Influenza (flu)

HPV vaccine (*Gardasil*)

Meningococcal vaccine (*Menactra, Menveo*)

Travel vaccines

Treatment history

All antiretroviral therapy (with start and stop dates for each drug)

Side effects and allergic reactions

Prophylaxis or treatment for opportunistic infections or complications

Other important information

Emergency contacts

Case manager or social worker

Advance directives (living will, durable power of attorney for health care)

HIV care is expensive. The average wholesale price of a year's worth of non-generic ART costs in the range of $28,000 to $35,000 per year, not including medical visits or lab tests.

employed, how much money you make, your immigration status, and whether you're disabled. Sadly, despite all these systems, some people fall through the cracks. Fortunately, having HIV has entitled you to benefits that would not be available if you had some other disease. In fact, I've written that the way we deliver HIV care would be a good model for a nationalized healthcare system for all!

HIV care is expensive. The average wholesale price of a year's worth of non-generic ART costs in the range of $28,000 to $35,000 per year, not including medical visits or lab tests. *Fortunately, almost no one has to pay this out of pocket—which is why it's critical to find out your options!* Those with private insurance are generally covered, though some plans require high copays or have limits on medication coverage. There may be government programs or pharmaceutical industry copay assistance programs that can help cover these costs; talk to your case manager or social worker.

If you're uninsured, or if your insurance doesn't cover your medications, you may qualify for the **AIDS Drug Assistance Program** (**ADAP**) in your state. (Massachusetts calls it "HIV Drug Assistance Program," or HDAP, just to be different.) This program provides HIV medications to people who fall below a specified income level. The coverage provided by ADAP programs varies from state to state. Some states' programs are quite generous, covering all medications, whereas others are skimpier and have shorter lists of covered medications. If you are using ADAP for your medication coverage, you must keep your paperwork up to date. Medical visits and lab tests are often paid for by federal **Ryan White Care Act** funds that are received by some HIV providers or treatment centers. Finally, the

AIDS Drug Assistance Program (ADAP)
A federally funded program that provides antiretroviral medications and other HIV-related medications to those who have no other way to pay for them.

Ryan White Care Act
A government-funded program that provides money on a state or local level to provide care for uninsured people with HIV.

ACA has made it easier for people with HIV to qualify for **Medicaid** or private insurance. In some states, Ryan White funds can be used to pay insurance premiums.

The complexities of insurance, benefits, and entitlements vary too much and change too quickly for me to be able to do them justice in this book. My advice is to talk to an HIV-savvy case manager or social worker, and find out where you stand. You can find them at HIV clinics and AIDS service organizations.

Medicaid

An insurance program funded by the federal and state governments that provides coverage for medical care to low-income, uninsured people.

MEDICAL CARE

PART FIVE

Getting Started

What does my CD4 count mean?

What is a resistance test, and when should I get one?

What vaccinations do I need?

More . . .

22. What does my CD4 count mean?

Your blood contains three kinds of cells: **red blood cells (RBCs)** (that's where the color comes from), white blood cells (WBCs), and **platelets**. WBCs are part of our immune system, protecting us from infections. **Lymphocytes** are a type of WBC, and the CD4 cell is a specific type of lymphocyte, the one HIV directly targets. So all CD4 cells are lymphocytes, and all lymphocytes are WBCs.

The CD4 count measures the health of your immune system. It should be checked when you are first diagnosed to assess the urgency of starting ART (Question 28). It also tells us whether you need certain medicines to prevent opportunistic infections (Question 60). This strategy is called **prophylaxis**, which means prevention.

Once you're on ART, the CD4 cell count will increase. This varies from person to person but is typically 100 to 200 cells of improvement in the first few years of treatment. However, some have an increase that is more than this, some that is less. There are no treatments *besides* ART that make the CD4 cell count increase reliably.

Once you're on ART, the viral load is a much more important measure of your response to therapy than the CD4 count. If your viral load is undetectable— the goal of therapy—it's unlikely that you would ever make any changes based on the CD4 count. A good response to ART is to have an undetectable (or *nearly* undetectable—more on this later!) viral load and a CD4 count above 500, which is roughly in the normal range. Once you're at or near this level, continuing to monitor the CD4 cell count is not necessary provided the viral load stays suppressed. You can ask your provider to check your CD4 count, but they should not make changes in your treatment based on changes in the result

The CD4 count can vary from day to day—even from hour to hour. It can drop temporarily when you're sick and can be affected by the way it's processed in the lab. Please don't pay too much attention to a single count, and don't get too worried or excited about a single count that's lower or higher respectively with previous counts. The trend over years is much more important. When in doubt, you can also look at the **CD4 percent**—the percentage of your lymphocytes that are CD4 cells. This number doesn't vary as much as the CD4 count, so if your CD4 count has changed but your CD4 percent hasn't, chances are it's not an important change. And remember that a high normal CD4 count is no better than a low normal CD4 count. Once it's above 500, it doesn't matter what the number is. In other words, don't panic when the CD4 count "falls" from 920 to 880— this is all part of normal variation!

CD4 percent

The percentage of your lymphocytes that are CD4 cells.

CD8 cells (or **CD8 lymphocytes** or **T-suppressor cells**) are also affected by HIV, and we know that having a higher ratio of CD4 cells to CD8 cells (CD4/CD8 ratio) is better than having a lower ratio. But we don't use these numbers to make treatment decisions because there's nothing you can do with the results other than to take ART. They're not recommended tests; all they do is make CD4 monitoring more expensive. If you have access to your own lab reports, you can also see how this also makes the reports much more complicated!

CD8 cells (CD8 lymphocytes or T-suppressor cells)

"Suppressor" cells that complete the immune response. They can also be "killer" cells that kill cancer cells and other cells that are infected by a virus.

23. What's a viral load?

The viral load (viral HIV RNA) measures the amount of HIV in your blood. It's a measure of the activity of the virus and of how well ART is working. It's also used, along with the CD4 count, to help decide the urgency of starting treatment.

The viral load can range from very low to very high. At the low end, our viral load tests can go down to 20 to 40 copies, depending on the specific test used. At the high end, all the tests go into the millions. It is highest during acute HIV (especially if a person has symptoms) and in people with advanced disease who aren't on treatment. When treatment is effective, the viral load should be suppressed (meaning below the lower limit of the test), which is also sometimes called "undetectable"—generally less than 20 to 40 in the tests that are most commonly used. Having a suppressed viral load doesn't mean there's no virus; it just means that the viral load is too low to be measured by standard blood tests. I will be using the terms suppressed and undetectable interchangeably to describe having a viral load less than 20 to 40, which is the goal of treatment.

Your viral load should be measured 2 to 4 weeks after starting or changing therapy and then routinely— usually every 3 to 4 months—until the result is less than 20 to 40. Regular measurements are especially important after starting treatment because that's how you know whether the drugs are working. If you've been on ART with an undetectable viral load for years, checking it every 6 months is plenty—in fact, some of my patients have been suppressed for so long that they check this yearly. They've earned the privilege of less frequent testing!

After starting therapy, the viral load should drop at least ten-fold [1 **log (logarithm)**] during the first month of therapy (e.g., from 100,000 to 10,000), and it should be undetectable within 3 to 6 months. People who start with a very high viral load might take longer to become suppressed than those with lower viral loads. The viral load will decline faster if you're taking an integrase inhibitor (Question 29), usually becoming undetectable within 1 to 2 months.

If your viral load is detectable once in a while, don't panic. It may just be a **blip**—a single viral load that's detectable at low levels (usually below 200). Blips can result from normal lab variation (no lab test is 100% accurate), so they're generally nothing to be alarmed about, provided you're taking your medications faithfully. We define treatment **failure** as a viral load that is *repeatedly* above 200. If you have been suppressed on ART for a while and get a result back that is low-level detectable between 50 to 200, your provider might ask you to come in and repeat the test sooner than usual. Most of the time this next test will be fine if you're still taking your medications—these treatments just don't suddenly fail for no reason!

24. What is a resistance test, and when should I get one?

Resistance tests tell you which drugs will work to treat your particular virus. Not all viruses respond to all medications. Resistance tests help choose the best drugs for treatment. Unlike CD4 counts and viral loads, resistance tests aren't ordered on a regular basis. They're ordered for only two reasons: to find out

---

Log (logarithm)

Another way of expressing viral load results. A viral load of 100,000 is a viral load of five logs; 10,000 is four logs; 1,000 is three logs. A tenfold change in viral load is a one-log change. For example, a drop in viral load from 100,000 to 1,000 is a "two-log drop."

Blip

A single detectable viral load with undetectable viral loads before and after. Usually below 200.

Failure

Loss of activity of ART. Includes virologic failure (repeatedly detectable viral load > 200 on therapy), immunologic failure (falling CD4 count on therapy), and clinical failure (worsening symptoms on therapy).

Resistance

The ability of the virus to replicate despite the presence of antiretroviral medications.

Genotype test

In HIV, a type of resistance test that looks for specific resistance mutations known to cause resistance to antiretroviral drugs. This is the most commonly ordered test.

Phenotype test

A type of resistance test that measures the ability of the virus to replicate in varying concentrations of antiretroviral drugs.

Mutations

Changes in the normal genetic make-up of an organism due to a mistake that occurs during reproduction. In the case of HIV, some mutations can cause resistance, allowing the virus to replicate in the presence of antiretroviral drugs.

Resistance tests tell you which drugs will work to treat your particular virus.

whether you were infected with resistant virus and to find out whether you've developed **resistance** if your treatment is failing.

You should be tested for resistance as soon as you're diagnosed with HIV. Your provider should also order a resistance test if you're failing therapy, to determine which drugs are no longer working and which drugs to use next.

There are two types of resistance tests: **genotype tests** and **phenotype tests**. Genotype tests look for **mutations** (changes) in the genes of the virus that cause resistance to specific drugs. Phenotype tests measure the virus's ability to replicate (multiply or reproduce) in the presence of drugs. Genotype tests are faster and cheaper and are almost always done today. Phenotype tests take longer and cost more, and sometimes are used if the mutations detected on the genotype are difficult to interpret.

Resistance tests aren't perfect. The lab may not be able to do the test if your viral load is below 500, and the tests are better at finding out which drugs *won't* work than which ones *will*. Bad news (evidence of resistance) is always believable, but you have to take good news (evidence of sensitivity to drugs) with a grain of salt. They can't always give you reliable information about drugs you've taken in the past because resistant virus may be present in reservoirs but no longer detectable. Don't ignore old resistance test results. If resistance was detected 5 years ago, it's still there—even if it doesn't show up on a test today.

There are additional resistance tests ordered in some situations. Because resistance tests were developed before the drugs called integrase inhibitors (Question 29) were available, many tests will not check for integrase resistance unless it is specifically ordered. The *GenoSure Archive* is a genotype test that can be ordered even if your viral load is < 500 or even suppressed. It looks for archived resistance: resistance you developed in the past that wouldn't necessarily be detected by standard resistance tests. Although we have little clinical experience with it so far, it has the potential to help guide the choice of therapy in people who don't have access to old medical records and resistance tests.

25. What other tests do I need?

Here's a list of important tests. Some are ordered just once, when you're first diagnosed, while others are ordered on a regular basis:

- **Complete blood count** (**CBC**). At baseline and every 3 to 6 months to look for anemia (**hemoglobin** and **hematocrit**), low white blood cell count, or platelet problems.

- **Comprehensive chemistry panel**. At baseline and every 3 to 6 months, mainly to assess the liver and kidneys.

- **Hepatitis** *tests*. Baseline testing for hepatitis A, B, and C and follow-up antibodies for A and B after vaccination to see if it worked (Questions 79 and 80). If the initial tests show evidence of either chronic hepatitis B or C, then you need further testing, including hepatitis B or C viral load tests (**HBV DNA** or **HCV RNA**). In injection drug users or gay men at high risk, HCV testing should be ordered on a regular basis.

GETTING STARTED

Complete blood count (CBC)

A standard blood test that measures the red and white blood cell counts, hematocrit, hemoglobin, and platelet count.

Hemoglobin

The oxygen-carrying component of red blood cells. Also used as a measure of the amount of red blood cells in the blood.

Hematocrit

A measure of the amount of red blood cells in the blood.

Comprehensive chemistry panel

A standard blood test that measures kidney function, looks for evidence of liver disease, assesses nutritional status, and looks for electrolyte (sodium, potassium) abnormalities.

Hepatitis

Inflammation or infection of the liver.

HBV DNA

The "viral load" for hepatitis B, used to make the diagnosis in some people with negative HBV antibodies and to monitor response to hepatitis B therapy.

HCV RNA

The "viral load" for hepatitis C, used to confirm the diagnosis in people with a positive HCV antibody, to make the diagnosis in some people with a negative antibody, and to monitor response to hepatitis C therapy.

Tuberculin skin test (TST, or purified protein derivative [PPD])

A skin test used to look for evidence of past exposure to *Mycobacterium tuberculosis*, the bacterium that causes tuberculosis. The most common form of TST is the PPD (purified protein derivative).

Interferon-gamma releasing assay (IGRA)

A blood test used to detect latent infection with the TB bacterium as an alternative to a tuberculin skin test. Two are available, QuantiFERON-TB Gold and T-SPOT.TB.

Toxoplasma IgG antibody

Serologic testing detects antibodies in the blood that are produced in response to an infection.

- *Tests for sexually transmitted infection.* Tests for syphilis, gonorrhea, and chlamydia at least once a year if you've been sexually active (Question 89).

- *Tuberculosis testing.* **Tuberculin skin test (TST)** with **purified protein derivative (PPD)**, or **interferon-gamma releasing assay (IGRA)** such as QuantiFERON-TB Gold or T-SPOT.TB to find out whether you have TB infection that needs preventive treatment (Question 59).

- **Toxoplasma IgG antibody.** To find out whether you've been exposed to the parasite that causes **toxoplasmosis** (Question 56).

- **Pap smear.** In women, to look for **cervical dysplasia** (changes in the cells of the cervix) or cancer. Pap smears should be repeated at least yearly. **Anal Pap smears** should be considered in both women and men, especially those who've had receptive anal sex (Question 81).

- **Fasting glucose** *and* **lipid panel.** Before starting ART and periodically after that, especially if you're on HIV drugs that increase cholesterol, triglycerides, and blood sugar (Question 43).

- **Urinalysis.** To look for kidney problems or signs of infection (Question 49). This test should be ordered every 6 months if you're taking a drug regimen that includes the older form of tenofovir, called tenofovir DF (*Viread, Truvada, Complera, Atripla,* or *Stribild*).

Other tests that are sometimes ordered include antibodies against CMV (anti-CMV IgG), a chest x-ray, and an HLA B*5701 assay, to find out whether it's safe to take abacavir (Question 45).

26. *What vaccinations do I need?*

- **Tetanus toxoid (dT or Tdap).** Everyone needs a tetanus booster every 10 years. If you haven't had the Tdap, which includes diphtheria and pertussis (whopping cough) vaccines, you need that once, and it's not necessary to wait until you're due for your next tetanus booster.

- **Pneumococcal vaccine.** These vaccines help protect you against **pneumococcus,** a bacterium that causes pneumonia. Start with *Prevnar 13,* followed at least 8 weeks later with two *Pneumovax* doses given 5 years apart. If you received the *Pneumovax* first, wait at least a year before receiving *Prevnar 13.*

- **Hepatitis A vaccine.** If you've never had **hepatitis A** and you're not immune to it (with a positive total or IgG **HAV antibody**), consider getting the two-shot vaccine series with follow-up antibody testing to be sure the vaccine worked. Hepatitis A vaccine is especially important for gay and bisexual men, travelers to resource-limited countries, and people who also have chronic hepatitis B or C.

- **Hepatitis B vaccine.** If you've never had hepatitis B and you're not immune to it (with a positive surface antibody [HBsAb]), you should get the three-part vaccine series with follow-up antibody testing to be sure the vaccine worked. There's also a three-dose combination vaccine (*Twinrix*) that protects you against both hepatitis A and B. A new hepatitis B vaccine called HEPLISAV might work for you if the original vaccine didn't.

- **Influenza ("flu")** *vaccine.* A flu shot* is recommended in the fall, not because HIV-positive people get more flu or worse flu than anyone else, but because it's awful getting the flu—and potentially

---

Toxoplasmosis

Disease caused by the parasite, *Toxoplasma gondii.*

Pap smear

A diagnostic test used to look for cervical dysplasia and cervical cancer. Now also being used to diagnose anal dysplasia (see **Anal Pap smear**).

Cervical dysplasia

Abnormal cells of the cervix, the mouth of the uterus, caused by human papillomavirus (HPV). If left untreated, it can progress to cervical cancer.

Anal Pap smear

A diagnostic test to screen for anal dysplasia. Also called "anal cytology."

Fasting glucose

Measures blood glucose levels after hours without food.

Lipid panel

A blood test that measures lipid levels in your blood (cholesterol and fats).

life threatening if you have other medical problems such as asthma or heart trouble. Get the injectable vaccine, not the live-virus nasal spray.

- **Varicella-zoster virus** *(chickenpox) vaccine.* If your CD4 count is above 200, you don't remember having ever had chickenpox or shingles, and you have a negative anti-varicella IgG antibody, consider getting this vaccine.

- *Shingles (herpes zoster) vaccine.* There are two versions of the vaccine. The newer version, called *Shingrix,* is more effective than the old *Zostavax* and the one to get if you're over 50. It is two doses, separated by 2 to 6 months.

*The flu shot doesn't cause the flu. It's typically given during cold season, so it's inevitable that some people will catch a cold shortly after getting vaccinated and will blame the vaccine. Don't be one of those people!

- **Human papillomavirus (HPV)** *vaccine.* The best time to get this vaccine is before you've ever had sex, but it's currently recommended for men and women up to the age of 26. The latest recommendation is that you can get it up to the age of 45 if you and your provider think you might still benefit. It prevents cancers caused by HPV, including cervical and anal cancer (Question 81). Even if you already have HPV-related conditions (anogenital warts, cervical or anal dysplasia), it may still protect you against strains you haven't been infected with. If you're over 26, you can still consider getting vaccinated, but it's less likely to be covered by your insurance.

- **Meningococcal vaccine.** There have been a number of cases and outbreaks of meningococcal disease, including meningitis, among gay men in various parts of the country. The meningococcal vaccine that covers serogroups C, W, and Y (MenACWY, *Menveo*, *Menactra*) is recommended. Two doses separated by at least 8 weeks is the schedule.

Vaccines for international travel are discussed in Question 93.

Vaccines work best when the immune system is strong. If you'll soon be starting ART, the vaccines will be more effective if you wait until after your CD4 count has risen and your viral load is undetectable.

Hepatitis A

A viral infection of the liver caused by hepatitis A virus (HAV).

HAV antibody

A blood test for hepatitis A.

Influenza ("flu")

A viral infection caused by influenza virus that causes fever, muscle aches, respiratory symptoms, and gastrointestinal symptoms. A bad cold is not the flu.

Varicella-zoster virus

The virus that causes chickenpox (primary varicella) and shingles (herpes zoster).

Human papillomavirus (HPV)

A sexually transmitted virus that causes abnormal cells (dysplasia) in the cervix, anus, and mouth, which can lead to cancer if not treated.

Meningococcal vaccine

A vaccine that prevents meningococcal disease.

PART SIX

Starting Treatment

How does antiretroviral therapy work?

How do my provider and I choose my first regimen?

Why is adherence so important?

More . . .

27. How does antiretroviral therapy work?

Antiretroviral drugs don't kill or cure HIV; they stop it from replicating (reproducing itself). If you stop replication, you stop the virus from infecting new cells. Suppressing replication also reduces the immune activation and inflammation that are thought to cause much of the damage to the immune system (Question 9). Turning off replication, immune activation, and inflammation allows the immune system to recover and the CD4 count to increase.

Combination therapy has been a guiding principle since the mid-1990s. The reason for combining several drugs into a single **regimen** (or "cocktail"—but don't use this term!) is to prevent resistance.

When the virus reproduces, it doesn't do so carefully. It's in a hurry and makes lots of mistakes, which are called mutations. Billions of **virions** (virus particles) are produced each day if you're not on therapy. Because of the high error rate, almost every mutation that *could* occur *does* occur, on a daily basis. Before the days of ART that could fully suppress replication, treatment for HIV involved one or two relatively weak drugs. Mutations that allowed the virus to replicate in the presence of those drugs could appear spontaneously. Those resistant mutants then had an advantage over the original **wild-type virus** (drug-sensitive virus without mutations). Over time, they became selected as the predominant **strain**, and the drugs were no longer effective.

It's far more difficult for the virus to spontaneously develop enough mutations to cause resistance to multiple drugs. Plus, when the viral load is suppressed, replication stops, and the virus needs to replicate to develop

Combination therapy

The use of more than one antiretroviral drug to suppress HIV.

Regimen

A combination of antiretroviral drugs.

Virions

Single virus particles.

Wild-type virus

The strain of HIV that occurs "in the wild"—without the presence of antiretroviral drugs that could select for mutations. Generally a non-mutant, drug-sensitive virus.

Strain

In the case of HIV, a type of virus, as in "drug-resistant strain."

new mutations. When you're taking an ART regimen that includes enough active drugs, resistance can only occur when drug levels aren't high enough to keep the virus from replicating, such as when you miss doses.

While most current ART regimens consist of at least three drugs, there's nothing magic about the number three. It's possible to use fewer drugs if they're potent enough to lead to viral suppression and if they have a high enough "resistance barrier," meaning that the virus needs multiple mutations to develop resistance.

Antiretroviral drugs don't kill HIV; they stop it from replicating (reproducing itself).

28. Should I start treatment?

Yes! Current U.S. guidelines recommend treatment for *everyone* with HIV, as the benefits to your health are clear, and treatment also prevents a person from spreading the virus to someone else.

What's different from person-to-person is the urgency of starting treatment. If you've already had a complication of HIV, or an AIDS diagnosis, or even just a CD4 cell count less than 200, you should start ART right now. The only exception to this rule is for people with an opportunistic infection called cryptococcal meningitis. In this condition, it's better to start treatment for this infection for a couple of weeks before starting ART. But this is the exception to the rule.

If you have HIV and are pregnant, you should also start ART now. This treatment prevents you from passing the virus on to your unborn baby.

What about if you're healthier and have a higher CD4 cell count? The benefits to you, and to others, still make starting ART worthwhile, and I recommend that you do it sooner rather than later. However, it is not an emergency. But what I've found is that when I discuss all the benefits of ART with my patients, they typically want to start the day I meet them—and this is fine! There is no medical reason why you should delay. In fact, some studies show that people with HIV are more likely to stay in care if they are prescribed ART at their first visit.

There are other reasons to start ART regardless of your CD4 count:

- *Hepatitis B.* Because you can treat both HIV and hepatitis B with the same drugs (Question 80).
- *HIV-associated nephropathy (HIVAN).* Because ART is the only effective treatment (Question 49).
- *Coronary heart disease (or high cardiac risk).* Because HIV increases your risk for heart disease (Question 47).
- *Risk of sexual transmission.* Because lowering your viral load makes you less infectious to others (Question 86).

There is only one group of people with HIV that ART has not been proven beneficial. Around one in a thousand people with HIV have no detectable viral load even without being on HIV treatment. For them, their immune system is doing the work of ART in controlling viral replication. Such people whose viral loads are undetectable without treatment are called **elite controllers,** or **non-viremic controllers**. Treatment of elite controllers may benefit them by reducing chronic inflammation and immune activation that could cause long-term complications. But since this benefit is still theoretical, I don't push too hard,

Elite controllers (or non-viremic controllers)

HIV-infected people whose CD4 counts remain high and whose viral loads are undetectable without treatment.

provided they have normal and stable CD4 counts. In my experience, some elite controllers have chosen to go on therapy, and others favor periodic monitoring. And it's very important that this monitoring occurs, because some people over time lose control of viral replication, and then definitely need to start therapy!

29. What are the classes of antiretroviral drugs, and why do they matter?

HIV goes through several stages in its life span, beginning with its entry into a human cell and ending with the release of new virus particles into the bloodstream that then infect new cells. This is called the viral life cycle (Figure 1). Antiretroviral drugs work by interfering with one of the stages of the life cycle, and they're classified based on which stage they inhibit. Talking about **drug classes** and life cycle stages gets a little technical, but learning it has some value. The drugs within a given class share some characteristics, such as how effective they are and side effects. Plus, if you're a science geek, it's kind of cool! The drugs are listed by category in **Table 3**.

1. **Entry** into the CD4 cell (**entry inhibitors**). This stage has three sub stages:

   a. **Attachment** of **gp120**, a portion of the **envelope** (the outer part of the virus) to the **CD4 receptor** on the surface of the CD4 cell. The only drug that blocks attachment is ibalizumab, a monoclonal antibody that binds to the CD4 receptor, blocking viral entry. Another drug called fostemsavir is in development.

STARTING TREATMENT

Drug classes

Categories or groups of HIV drugs that are classified by the way the drugs work and the stage of the viral life cycle that they target.

Entry

The process by which HIV enters human cells.

Entry inhibitors

Drugs that block entry of the virus into the CD4 cell.

Antiretroviral drugs work by interfering with one of the stages of the life cycle, and they're classified based on which stage they inhibit.

Attachment

The first stage of entry, in which the virus binds to the CD4 receptor. Attachment inhibitors would block this step, though none is currently approved.

Table 3 Coformulated Single-Tablet Regimens (Last updated July 10, 2019; last reviewed July 10, 2019)

The following table includes dose recommendations for FDA-approved STR products. Drugs listed in this table are arranged in alphabetical order by trade name within each section.

Trade Name (Abbreviations)	ARV Drugs Included in the STR	Dosing Recommendation
INSTI plus Two NRTIs		
Biktarvy (BIC/TAF/FTC)	Bictegravir 50 mg/tenofovir alafenamide 25 mg/emtricitabine 200 mg	One tablet once daily
Genvoya (EVG/c/TAF/FTC)	Elvitegravir 150 mg/cobicistat 150 mg/tenofovir alafenamide 10 mg/emtricitabine 200 mg	One tablet once daily with food
Stribild (EVG/c/TDF/FTC)	Elvitegravir 150 mg/cobicistat 150 mg/tenofovir disoproxil fumarate 300 mg/emtricitabine 200 mg	One tablet once daily with food
Triumeq (DTG/ABC/3TC)	Dolutegravir 50 mg/abacavir 600 mg/lamivudine 300 mg	One tablet once daily
INSTI plus One NRTI		
Dovato (DTG/3TC)	Dolutegravir 50 mg/lamivudine 300 mg	One tablet once daily
PI plus Two NRTIs		
Symtuza (DRV/c/TAF/FTC)	Darunavir 800 mg/cobicistat 150 mg/tenofovir alafenamide 10 mg/emtricitabine 200 mg	One tablet once daily with food
NNRTI plus Two NRTIs		
Atripla (EFV/TDF/FTC)	Efavirenz 600 mg/tenofovir disoproxil fumarate 300 mg/emtricitabine 200 mg	One tablet once daily on an empty stomach, preferably at bedtime
Complera (RPV/TDF/FTC)	Rilpivirine 25 mg/tenofovir disoproxil fumarate 300 mg/emtricitabine 200 mg	One tablet once daily with a meal
Delstrigo (DOR/TDF/3TC)	Doravirine 100 mg/tenofovir disoproxil fumarate 300 mg/lamivudine 300 mg	One tablet once daily

Trade Name (Abbreviations)	ARV Drugs Included in the STR	Dosing Recommendation
Odefsey (RPV/TAF/FTC)	Rilpivirine 25 mg/tenofovir alafenamide 25 mg/emtricitabine 200 mg	One tablet once daily with a meal
Symfi (EFV/TDF/3TC)	Efavirenz 600 mg/tenofovir disoproxil fumarate 300 mg/lamivudine 300 mg	One tablet once daily on an empty stomach, preferably at bedtime
Symfi Lo (EFV/TDF/3TC)	Efavirenz 400 mg/tenofovir disoproxil fumarate 300 mg/lamivudine 300 mg	One tablet once daily on an empty stomach, preferably at bedtime
INSTI plus One NNRTI		
Juluca (DTG/RPV)	Dolutegravir 50 mg/rilpivirine 25 mg	One tablet once daily with a meal

Key: 3TC = lamivudine; ABC = abacavir; ARV = antiretroviral; BIC = bictegravir; c = cobicistat; DOR = doravirine; DRV = darunavir; DTG = dolutegravir; EFV = efavirenz; EVG = elvitegravir; FDA = Food and Drug Administration; FTC = emtricitabine; INSTI = integrase strand transfer inhibitor; NNRTI = non-nucleoside reverse transcriptase inhibitor; NRTI = nucleoside reverse transcriptase inhibitor; PI = protease inhibitor; RPV = rilpivirine; STR = single-tablet regimen; TAF = tenofovir alafenamide; TDF = tenofovir disoproxil fumarate

b. Binding of coreceptors to gp120. There are two **coreceptors** (or **chemokines**) on the cell surface—CCR5 and CXCR4. Maraviroc (*Selzentry*) is a drug that blocks CCR5 (**CCR5 antagonist**). We don't have any drugs that block CXCR4 attachment. Before using a CCR5 inhibitor, you need a special blood test called a **tropism assay** to make sure you have **R5 virus** (virus that enters the cell using only the CCR5 coreceptor). If some of your virus gets in through CXCR4 (**X4** or **dual/mixed [D/M] virus**), maraviroc will not work.

c. **Fusion** (merging) of the coating of the virus with the surface of the CD4 cell, which

gp120

The part of the envelope (outer surface) of HIV that binds to receptors on the surface of the CD4 cell, allowing entry into the cell.

Envelope

The outer surface of the HIV virus.

CD4 receptor

A protein on the surface of the CD4 cell that the virus attaches to before entering the cell.

61

allows the genetic material (RNA) of the virus to enter the cell. Enfuvirtide (T-20, *Fuzeon*) is an approved injectable drug that's rarely used since our current treatments are much easier to take.

2. **Reverse transcription** turns viral RNA into DNA. It's called "reverse" because it's the opposite of normal transcription, which turns DNA into RNA. This process requires reverse transcriptase (RT), an enzyme (protein) that's brought into the cell from the virus. There are two types of reverse transcriptase inhibitors:

a. **Nucleoside analog reverse transcriptase inhibitors** (or **NRTIs** or **"nukes"**) mimic the normal building blocks of DNA. They get inserted into the growing DNA chain, but because they're not the right nucleosides, they interfere with the process, stopping the DNA chain from being formed.

b. **Non-nucleoside reverse transcriptase inhibitors** (**NNRTIs**) stop the same process, but they do it by binding directly to the reverse transcriptase enzyme, preventing it from doing its dirty work.

3. **Integration** is the insertion of the newly created viral DNA into the human DNA in the cell's nucleus. This step requires a viral enzyme called **integrase**. **Integrase inhibitors** prevent integrase from doing its job. They are sometimes called "integrase strand transfer inhibitors," abbreviated INSTIs.

4. **Protease** inhibitors (PIs) block a late stage in the viral life cycle in which proteins created from viral DNA are cut to create the building blocks of the new viral particles.

Coreceptors (or chemokines)

Proteins on the surface of the CD4 cell and other cells that the virus binds to after attaching to the CD4 receptor but before entering the cell. There are two coreceptors: CCR5 and CXCR4.

CCR5 antagonist

A drug that blocks CCR5.

Tropism assay

A blood test used to find out whether your virus enters the CD4 cell using the CCR5 coreceptor (R5 virus) or the CXCR4 coreceptor (X4 virus) or both coreceptors. This test is necessary before taking a CCR5 inhibitor, which should only be used with R5 virus.

R5 virus

HIV that enters the CD4 cell using the CCR5 coreceptor. This type of virus can be treated with CCR5 inhibitors (see **Coreceptor**).

X4 or dual/mixed (D/M) virus

HIV that enters the CD4 cell using the CXCR4 coreceptor, or both receptors. X4 virus cannot be treated with CCR5 inhibitors.

5. Maturation inhibitors are somewhat like protease inhibitors, but they block the cleavage of viral proteins in a different way. There is a maturation inhibitor in development.

30. How do my provider and I choose my first regimen?

Answering a question like this in a book is challenging, because my answer may be out of date by the time you read it. Things change fast as new drugs are developed and new data emerge. The Appendix lists a number of resources that can help keep you up to date.

First, make sure you've had a baseline resistance test (Question 24) before starting your regimen. You don't want to take a drug that will not work because of resistance. Besides being a waste of time and money, it could put you at risk of developing resistance to the other drugs in your regimen. If you are starting a recommended regimen that includes 2 NRTIs and an INSTI, you do not need to wait for the results to return before starting.

Your provider needs to know some things about you to help determine the best regimen. What other medical conditions do you have? What medications do you take? Do you have any big travel plans or events coming up? Are your kidneys and liver in good shape? What's your daily schedule like? Do you eat regular meals? Are you worried that you might miss doses or stop therapy periodically? If you're a woman, is there a possibility of pregnancy?

There are also questions that you need to ask your provider, nurse, or pharmacist before you start. Should I

Fusion

The final stage of entry in which the envelope of the virus fuses (merges) with the membrane of the cell, allowing entry of the virus into the cells. A fusion inhibitor blocks this process.

Reverse transcription

The conversion of viral RNA into DNA by reverse transcriptase. (Normal transcription involves the conversion of DNA into RNA.)

Nucleoside analog reverse transcriptase inhibitors (or NRTIs, or "nukes")

A class of antiretroviral drugs that blocks reverse transcription of viral RNA into DNA by mimicking nucleosides, the normal building blocks of DNA.

Non-nucleoside reverse transcriptase inhibitors (NNRTIs)

A class of antiretroviral drugs that blocks reverse transcription of viral RNA into DNA by interfering with the activity of reverse transcriptase.

Integration

The insertion of viral DNA into human DNA in the nucleus of the cell.

Integrase

A viral enzyme that allows integration (insertion) of viral DNA into human DNA.

Integrase inhibitor

An antiretroviral drug that blocks the integration process. These are often abbreviated INSTI, standing for "integrase strand transfer inhibitor."

take my meds with food or without? Does the time of day I take the meds matter? How do I get refills? What if I'm late for a dose (Question 31)? If I run out of one medication, should I still take the others? What side effects can I expect, and what should I do if I get certain side effects (Question 32)? Don't start therapy until your questions have been answered.

Table 4 lists the advantages and disadvantages of the various drugs, combination pills, and single-tablet regimens. The recommended and alternative starting regimens all include either an NNRTI, a protease inhibitor (PI), or an integrase inhibitor (sometimes abbreviated INSTI for "integrase strand transfer inhibitor" because "II" sounds and looks too weird). These agents are almost always used in combination with two NRTIs, which are sometimes called the "nuke backbone," though I don't like that term, since all components of a regimen are important. The only option for initial therapy that doesn't use three active drugs is dolutegravir plus lamivudine, which comes in a single tablet. There is not enough experience with this yet to make it a first-line recommended regimen, but it's the best choice if you can't take tenofovir or abacavir.

For many years, the two recommended NRTI pairs have been tenofovir/emtricitabine and abacavir/lamivudine. There are now two forms of tenofovir: the original tenofovir disoproxil fumarate (TDF) and the newer tenofovir alafenamide (TAF). TDF can sometimes

Table 4 Advantages and Disadvantages of Antiretroviral Drugs and Regimens for Initial Therapy. All recommended and alternative initial regimens consist of a pair of nucleoside reverse transcriptase inhibitors plus a third active agent from a different class. The one exception is lamivudine plus dolutegravir, which is an alternative regimen for people who cannot take either abacavir or tenofovir. Drugs that are no longer recommended because of side effects or other problems are not listed.

A. Nucleoside reverse transcriptase inhibitor (NRTI) pairs			
Drug or Drugs	**Forms and Brand Names**	**Advantages**	**Disadvantages**
Abacavir/ lamivudine (ABC/3TC)	*Epzicom* or generic and part of *Triumeq* (ABC/3TC/DTG)	No kidney or bone toxicity Coformulated with DTG as a recommended initial regimen	Must pre-test with HLA B*5701 to avoid ABC hypersensitivity reaction Less effective than TDF/FTC when combined with EFV or ATV/r in people with viral loads above 100,000 May increase risk of heart attack Unlike tenofovir-based combinations, not sufficient for treatment of hepatitis B
Tenofovir AF/ emtricitabine (TAF/FTC)	*Descovy*, and part of *Genvoya*, *Odefsey*, *Biktarvy*, and *Symtuza*	Less kidney and bone toxicity than tenofovir DF A recommended initial NRTI pair with several third agents Can be used to treat both HIV and hepatitis B	Does not lower lipids like tenofovir DF Will be more expensive than tenofovir DF/FTC when that becomes generic People receiving TAF/FTC-containing regimens gain more weight than those on TDF/FTC-containing regimens
Tenofovir DF/ emtricitabine (TDF/FTC)	*Truvada* and part of *Atripla*, *Complera*, and *Stribild* (TDF/FTC/ EVG/c)	Lowers lipid levels Can be used to treat both HIV and hepatitis B	Can cause kidney problems, especially in people with other risks for kidney disease (diabetes, high blood pressure) Causes more loss of bone density than other drugs
Tenofovir DF/ lamivudine (3TC)	Generic and part of *Delstrigo*	Less expensive than TDF/FTC and TAF/FTC	Similar to TDF/FTC

(continued)

Table 4 Advantages and Disadvantages of Antiretroviral Drugs and Regimens for Initial Therapy (*continued*)

B. Nonnucleoside reverse transcriptase inhibitors (NNRTIs)			
Drug	**Forms and Brand Names**	**Advantages**	**Disadvantages**
Doravirine (DOR)	*Pifeltro* and part of *Delstrigo*	Less rash and fewer central nervous system side effects than efavirenz Fewer drug interactions than rilpivirine Favorable lipid profile Can be taken with or without food Different resistance profile compared with other NNRTI Available as a STR (Delstrigo)	Not available with TAF/FTC as an STR Not tested in clinical trials against an integrase inhibitor
Efavirenz (EFV)	*Sustiva* or *generic*, and as part of *Symfi* or *Symfi Lo*	Was part of the first STR, so extensive clinical experience globally Remains in blood for a long time, so "forgiving" of missed doses Retains activity even a high viral loads	Can cause neurologic or psychiatric side effects, especially in the first few weeks, but long-term effects can also occur Can cause rash Resistance common if treatment fails Most common form of transmitted resistance is to efavirenz No TAF version available
Etravirine (ETR)	*Intelence*	Often active even when there is resistance to EFV and NVP Can be dissolved in water for those who cannot swallow pills	Not recommended for initial therapy Many drug interactions Tablet formulation is gritty, difficult for some to swallow

Drug	Forms and Brand Names	Advantages	Disadvantages
Nevirapine (NVP)	*Viramune*, *Viramune* XR, or generic	Inexpensive	Can cause severe liver toxicity or skin rash during first few weeks, especially in women with pre-treatment CD4 counts above 250 or men with counts above 400 Resistance common if treatment fails
Rilpivirine (RPV)	*Edurant* and as part of *Complera*, *Odefsey*, or *Juluuca*	Less rash and fewer neurologic side effects than EFV Does not raise lipids as much as EFV	Must be taken with a meal Can't be taken with proton pump inhibitors and other drugs used to treat reflux and ulcers Resistance common if treatment fails Not as effective if viral load > 100,000 or CD4 cell count < 200

C. Protease inhibitors (PIs). All should be given with the "boosters" ritonavir or cobicistat.

Atazanavir (ATV) plus ritonavir (RTV) or atazanavir/cobicistat (c)	*Reyataz* or *Evotaz* (ATV/c)	Resistance uncommon with failure Only PI not linked to increased risk of cardiovascular disease	Many drug interactions Can cause jaundice Should be taken with food Can cause kidney stones, gall stones, or kidney trouble

(continued)

67

Table 4 Advantages and Disadvantages of Antiretroviral Drugs and Regimens for Initial Therapy (*continued*)

Drug or drugs	Forms and Brand Names	Advantages	Disadvantages
Darunavir(DRV) plus ritonavir or darunavir/ cobicistat (c)	*Prezista* or *Prezcobix* (DRV/c) and part of *Symtuza*	Best tolerated PI Resistance unlikely with failure Only PI available as a single tablet regimen (Symtuza, TAF/FTC/DRV/c)	Many drug interactions Should be taken with food May cause rash May increase cardiovascular risk
Lopinavir/ritonavir (LPV/RTV)	*Kaletra* or generic	None	Many drug interactions Highest risk of GI side effects Increases lipids more than ATV or DRV May increase risk of cardiovascular disease

D. Integrase strand transfer inhibitors (INSTIs)

Drug or drugs	Forms and Brand Names	Advantages	Disadvantages
Bictegravir (BIC)	*Biktarvy* (TAF/FTC/BIC)	Few side effects Few drug interactions Higher barrier to resistance than RAL or EVG Only unboosted INSTI with tenofovir as part of a STR	Raises serum creatinine (but does not damage kidneys) Associated with more weight gain than non-INSTI based regimens Cannot use with active TB since rifampin lowers levels

Drug	Forms and Brand Names	Advantages	Disadvantages
Dolutegravir (DTG)	*Tivicay* or part of *Triumeq* or *Juluuca* or *Dovato*	Few side effects Few drug interactions Higher barrier to resistance than RAL or EVG Can be used with active TB (dose doubled with rifampin) Two-drug regimens of DTG/RPV (Juluuca) and DTG/3TC (Dovato) both options for people who cannot take ABC or tenofovir	Raises serum creatinine (but does not damage kidneys) Associated with more weight gain than non-INSTI based regimens DTG increases metformin levels, may require dose reduction DTG/3TC not tested in people with baseline viral loads > 500,000 DTG/RPV only approved for switch therapy, not initial treatment
Elvitegravir (EVG)	Part of *Stribild* or *Genvoya*	Few side effects Better tolerated than EFV	Many drug interactions Should be taken with food Increases serum creatinine (but does not damage kidneys) Resistance barrier lower than BIC and DTG
Raltegravir (RAL)	*Isentress* or *Isentress HD*	Few side effects Few drug interactions	Two pills No coformulation available Resistance barrier lower than BIC and DTG

Protease

A viral enzyme that cuts large viral proteins into smaller proteins, which are then used to create new virus particles. A protease inhibitor (PI) is an antiretroviral drug that blocks this process.

HLA B*5701

A blood test used to predict the likelihood of the abacavir hypersensitivity reaction (HSR), which is a severe allergic reaction. If the test is positive, you shouldn't take abacavir. If it's negative, you're extremely unlikely to develop HSR.

Clinical trial

A study in which a treatment for a medical condition is tested in human volunteers to determine the safety and/or effectiveness of the treatment.

cause kidney damage and/or loss of bone density, which doesn't seem to happen with TAF. For that reason, TAF/emtricitabine (*Descovy*, and part of *Biktarvy*, *Genvoya* and *Odefsey*) is replacing TDF/emtricitabine (*Truvada*, and part of *Stribild*, *Complera*, and *Atripla*). There is controversy about whether abacavir increases the risk of heart attack, which is mainly an issue for people who have a lot of cardiac risk factors already. You need an **HLA B*5701** test before taking any regimen containing abacavir (*Ziagen, Epivir, Trizivir, Triumeq*), since it can cause a serious allergic reaction in those who test positive—so serious that some people have needed hospitalization, or even died! So make sure you get that test if your provider wants to use abacavir. In people with viral loads above 100,000, *Epzicom* was less effective than *Truvada* in combination with some third agents, but that doesn't apply when it's combined with dolutegravir (usually in the form of *Triumeq*).

As for third agents, INSTIs have become the preferred way to start based on their outstanding safety and tolerability in **clinical trials**, with effectiveness that's at least as good as the PIs or NNRTIs and sometimes better. Raltegravir (*Isentress*) was the first INSTI, and although it's an excellent drug, it is two pills on its own and is not available in a single-tablet regimen (STR). Raltegravir has few drug interactions, an advantage for some people who are taking multiple medications. *Stribild* and *Genvoya* are STRs that combine elvitegravir (an INSTI), cobicistat (a drug that boosts elvitegravir levels), and the NRTI combination of TDF/emtricitabine (*Stribild*) or TAF/emtricitabine (*Genvoya*). They're well tolerated and effective, although cobicistat has drug interactions that are similar to those of ritonavir (*Norvir*) (Question 34). Because it contains TAF, *Genvoya* is rapidly replacing *Stribild*. Cobicistat is available as a standalone product (*Tybost*), but it's not often used.

Dolutegravir (*Tivicay*) and bictegravir are often called "second-generation" INSTIs to distinguish them from raltegravir and elvitegravir. They both have a higher barrier to resistance than those earlier drugs. This means that if people take them irregularly as part of a combination regimen, resistance is *much* less likely to happen with dolutegravir and bictegravir than raltegravir and elvitegravir. Dolutegravir can be prescribed with *Descovy* or *Truvada* or as an STR with ABC and 3TC (*Triumeq*) or just 3TC (Dovato). Bictegravir is co-formulated with tenofovir AF and emtricitabine as the single tablet regimen *Biktarvy*.

Even though INSTIs (in particular dolutegravir and bictegravir) have become the default third drugs to use with an NRTI pair, they are not perfect. Some people experience a headache or insomnia when taking INSTIs. And while all people with HIV gain weight when they start treatment—likely because their health is improving—people taking INSTI-based treatment appear to gain the most weight. It's not clear yet why this happens, and whether weight gain is simply the absence of side effects such as nausea or due to a direct effect of INSTIs on appetite.

Among the NNRTIs, efavirenz (*Sustiva*, and in combination with TDF/FTC as *Atripla*) had been the favored NNRTI for years because of its long-term safety and effectiveness in many clinical trials. Unfortunately, it causes "neuropsychiatric" side effects—dizziness, vivid dreams, nightmares, fuzzy thinking, and "brain fog"—during the first few days or weeks (Question 52). Some side effects can be longer lasting, including depression. As a result, it's becoming less popular given all the other regimens that don't take getting used to. In addition, there is no TAF-containing version of *Atripla*, which is another disadvantage of this combination. Doravirine (Pifeltro) is the newest drug in the NNRTI class, and has fewer side effects than efavirenz. It comes co-formulated with TDF/3TC as a single tablet regimen (*Delstrigo*). Rilpivirine (*Edurant*, and in combination with TAF/FTC as *Odefsey* and with TDF/FTC as *Complera* or *Eviplera*, depending on the country you live in) is better tolerated than efavirenz, but it has to be taken with a meal, and you can't take it with drugs such as proton pump inhibitors that are used to treat heartburn, reflux, and ulcers. Nevirapine (*Viramune*) has fallen out of favor, mainly because it can have severe early side effects in people who start therapy with high CD4 counts. Delavirdine (*Rescriptor*) is no longer recommended, and etravirine (*Intelence*) is generally not used for initial therapy.

Boosted protease inhibitors

These combine a protease inhibitor (PI) with cobicistat or with a low dose of ritonavir (*Norvir*), another PI that is used only to increase drug levels and prolong the half-life of other PIs.

PIs today are virtually always given as a **boosted protease inhibitor**, either with low doses of ritonavir (*Norvir*), a PI that's much too toxic to use at full dose, or with cobicistat (*Tybost* or included in *Prezcobix* and *Reyataz*). These pharmacoenhancers or "boosters" increase drug levels of the PIs, increasing their potency and allowing you to take them less often or with fewer pills. A clear advantage of boosted PI regimens is that they're virtually resistance-proof, making them good choices for people who aren't good at taking medications faithfully. (That advantage only applies to PIs, but not to the cobicistat-boosted elvitegravir contained in *Genvoya* and *Stribild*.) However, dolutegravir (*Tivcay*, and included in *Triumeq*) and bictegravir (included in *Biktarvy*) have the same advantage with fewer side effects and drug interactions. The favored PI for initial therapy is darunavir (*Prezista*), with atazanavir (*Reyataz*) coming in second because it was not quite as well tolerated in a large comparative trial. Both drugs are available in combination with cobicistat, as *Evotaz* and *Prezcobix*, so it's no longer necessary to take separate doses of *Norvir*. There's little reason to use any of the older PIs anymore.

31. Why is adherence so important?

Adherence (or **compliance**) is the word we use to describe your ability to "stick to" treatment recommendations, including taking medications and keeping clinic appointments. Adherence is important for any medical treatment, but it's *especially* important for HIV because of the risk of drug resistance. If you were non-adherent with your blood pressure medications, you might damage your heart, kidneys, or vision, but the drugs would still work once you started taking them properly. No matter how bad you are at keeping diabetes under control, insulin will work when it's taken. In contrast, HIV is a living organism whose sole reason for living is to replicate (reproduce itself). ART stops that replication. Missed doses and interruptions in treatment allow drug levels to fall. If they fall low enough, the virus starts replicating again. When it does, resistant mutants—virus particles that can replicate in the presence of drugs—have an advantage over the drug-sensitive strains. They can eventually replace the non-resistant (wild-type) virus as the dominant viral strain.

For a particularly vivid analogy that you won't soon forget, imagine a can full of the creatures from your nightmares: rats, cockroaches, spiders, or snakes—your choice. If you keep the lid on the can, the critters can't get out. But if you leave the lid ajar, the strongest will escape. They'll hook up with the other strong escapees, breeding super-creatures that you won't want to have

Adherence (or compliance)

The term used to refer to a patient's behavior with respect to following treatment recommendations, including taking medications, keeping medical appointments, etc.

around. Adherence to ART is the lid on the can. Keep it tightly closed!

Studies show that your ability to adhere to therapy has little to do with your race, sex, education level, or socioeconomic status. Things that *do* affect adherence are mental illness (including depression), drug or alcohol abuse, memory problems, and a chaotic lifestyle. If any of those issues apply to you, address them before starting therapy (**Part 13**). People are more likely to adhere if they understand why they're on treatment, why adherence is important, and if they participated in the decision to start treatment. Finally, it helps to have what is called "self-efficacy": the confidence that you have the ability to affect your future by completing actions you take in the present.

Fortunately, adherence is easier now because the available regimens are better tolerated, are usually taken just once day, and typically consist of 1 to 2 pills. The newer drugs have longer **half-lives** than the older drugs, which means they last a long time in the blood. That gives you more "wiggle room" in the timing of doses. But missing doses or interrupting treatment is still risky, especially with NNRTIs and some INSTIs because it only takes a single mutation to get high-level resistance. If you're worried about your ability to adhere to therapy, talk to your provider, nurse, or pharmacist before you start therapy. Many HIV clinics have programs that can help with adherence.

Half-life

The amount of time it takes for the blood levels of a drug to decline by 50% after the last dose. Drugs with longer half-lives remain in the blood longer and can be taken less often.

Here are a few tips to help you adhere:

1. Get a pillbox from the pharmacy—one that has labeled compartments for each day and dose. Put your pills in it each week, even if you're

only taking one pill per day. You'll never have to wonder whether you took your pills or not—if they're still in the box, you didn't.

2. Link your doses to something else you do *every* day—eating a meal, brushing your teeth, or making coffee. If you have a cup of coffee every morning, put your pills beside the coffee maker so you see them when you reach for your morning cup.

3. Always check your medication supply, and order your refills in advance—don't run out on weekends or holidays. If you're using a mail-order pharmacy, you have to plan even further ahead.

4. Talk to your provider or pharmacist about what to do if you forget a dose. With most HIV drugs, it's OK to take them as soon as you remember, or even to double the next dose, but I wouldn't suggest doubling the dose of efavirenz (*Sustiva, Atripla*) because of the side effects you're likely to experience.

My patients who do best are the ones who are a little obsessive-compulsive about taking their medications. When I ask, "How many doses have you missed since I saw you last?" they look at me as if I have suddenly grown a second head!

32. What if I have side effects?

I'll been using two terms—**side effects** and **toxicity**, which are not always the same thing. Side effects can make your life unpleasant, but they don't always mean that the drugs are hurting you (for example, nervous system side effects from efavirenz, discussed in

Side effects

Undesirable effects of a medication or treatment that are noticeable to the person being treated (see **Toxicity**).

Toxicity

Damage to the body caused by a drug or other substance.

Pancreatitis

Inflammation of the pancreas, resulting in abdominal pain, loss of appetite, nausea, and vomiting. Can be fatal.

Hypersensitivity reactions (HSRs)

Reactions, often allergic, to a medication or other substance.

Starting therapy is sometimes a trial-and-error process. You may end up on a different combination than the one you started on. Substituting one drug for another because of side effects is fine.

Question 52). On the other hand, you may feel fine even though you're taking a drug that's causing toxicity (for example, high cholesterol from some PIs, Question 43). Finally, you may have a side effect that's also a toxicity, such as painful feet caused by nerve damage from stavudine (Questions 45 and 52), which fortunately is a drug we don't use anymore.

Because you'll be starting at a combination of new medications at once, it's not unusual to experience side effects. Side effects and toxicities of specific drugs are discussed in **Part 8**. Some side effects, such as the nervous system side effects of efavirenz or upset stomach with zidovudine, are worst when you first start treatment, and then get better as your body becomes used to the medication. Others are chronic but manageable, such as loose stools with PIs. Some can be acute and serious, such as **pancreatitis** with didanosine or **hypersensitivity reactions** (**HSRs**) with abacavir or nevirapine. Other side effects can get worse with continued use (nerve damage with stavudine) or can cause a risk of long-term problems (high cholesterol or blood sugar due to some PIs, which increase the risk of heart disease). Fortunately, *none* of the drugs I've just mentioned is a recommended drug that's commonly used today. Today's drugs are a lot safer than the older ones.

Starting therapy is sometimes a trial-and-error process. You may end up on a different combination than the one you started on. Substituting one drug for another because of side effects is fine, and is much safer than stopping completely and starting over later, which can increase the risk of resistance. When starting your first regimen, it's important to know how to contact your provider if you have unexpected side effects or side effects that you can't put up with until your next visit.

33. How should my treatment be monitored?

Once you start ART, it's important to get lab tests done frequently—usually every month or so at the beginning. The purpose of monitoring is to make sure you're responding to the medications appropriately and not developing toxicity.

The best measure of response to therapy is your viral load. It should decrease at least tenfold in the first month, which means that if it started out at 100,000, it should be well below 10,000. Your viral load should then continue to fall until it becomes undetectable (less than 20), usually within 4 to 6 months. Integrase inhibitors will lower the viral load much faster—often within 1 to 2 months. That doesn't necessarily make them better, but it's still gratifying. I generally check the viral load every 4 to 6 weeks until it becomes undetectable, then every 3 to 4 months after that. In my patients who have had undetectable viral loads for many years, I often switch to a 6-month schedule.

The CD4 count will also increase on therapy, but the amount of increase is impossible to predict. Starting with a low CD4 count, having a low baseline viral load, having hepatitis C, or being older can all blunt the CD4 response to therapy. In the past, we always ordered a CD4 count every time we checked the viral load, but that's no longer recommended because the viral load is so much more important. Once your viral load is undetectable and your CD4 count is high and stable, it becomes an optional test.

We look for drug toxicity with standard blood tests. The complete blood count (CBC) measures the red and white blood cell counts and the platelet count. The only antiretroviral medication that's likely to affect these counts is zidovudine (AZT), which can cause **anemia** (low red blood cell count). A comprehensive chemistry panel includes measurements of kidney function, liver health, and blood sugar. A urinalysis should be checked twice a year if you're taking a regimen that includes tenofovir DF (*Viread, Truvada, Complera, Atripla,* and *Stribild*). You should get a fasting lipid panel and blood sugar at least once a year, especially if you're taking medications that have metabolic side effects.

Anemia

A deficiency of red blood cells, usually diagnosed by a low hemoglobin or hematocrit on a complete blood count.

34. Can my HIV drugs interact with other medications?

They sure can, which is why you should always carry a list of all of the medicines you're taking and show the list to other providers who are treating you. The PIs, NNRTIs, cobicistat, and CCR5 antagonists are the drugs most likely to interact with other medications, and also with each other. There are few interactions with NRTIs, fusion inhibitors, raltegravir, dolutegravir, or bictegravir. Listing all drug interactions here would be impossible, but I'll make a few points about interactions that are especially common and important:

Statins

The common name for HMG CoA reductase inhibitors, drugs that lower cholesterol.

- *Statins.* The levels of the **statins** (drugs that lower cholesterol) can be increased by ritonavir (*Norvir*) and cobicistat (*Tybost, Prezcobix, Evotaz*), causing muscle breakdown and kidney failure. Some, such as simvastatin (*Zocor*) and lovastatin (*Mevacor*), should *never* be used with PIs or cobicistat. Others, such as atorvastatin (*Lipitor*), pravastatin (*Pravachol*), and rosuvastatin (*Crestor*), can generally be used at low doses, though pravastatin—a weaker statin—should be avoided with darunavir (*Prezista,*

Prezcobix). A newer agent, pitavastatin (*Livalo*), has no important drug interactions.

- *Birth control pills.* PIs, NNRTIs, and cobicistat can lower drug levels, making them less effective, so you may need to use another method of birth control if you're taking one of these drugs.

- *Rifampin.* **Rifampin** is a drug used to treat TB and some bacterial infections. It affects the levels of most PIs and NNRTIs. It shouldn't be taken with TAF (*Descovy, Genvoya, Odefsey*) or with any PI or NNRTI except efavirenz. If you're using nevirapine or PIs, rifabutin can be used as an alternative.

Rifampin
A drug used to treat tuberculosis and some other bacterial infections.

- *Steroid sprays.* PIs and cobicistat can increase steroid levels with fluticasone, a common ingredient in nasal sprays or inhalers (*Flonase, Advair, Flovent*). Use alternatives if possible. This interaction is also a problem with steroids that are injected into joints to treat pain.

- *Narcotics.* Methadone levels are decreased by some NNRTIs and PIs, which can cause withdrawal. Fentanyl levels can be increased, resulting in overdose.

- *Proton pump inhibitors* (PPIs).* These drugs, used to treat acid reflux and ulcers, should generally not be used with atazanavir (*Reyataz, Evotaz*) or rilpivirine (*Edurant, Complera, Eviplera, Odefsey*), because the PPIs can lower the HIV drugs' absorption so that you get less than the dose you need. If you have to take a PPI with one of these drugs, it should be at the lowest dose and with careful dose separation. Other drugs that lower stomach acid,

Carry a list of all of the medicines you're taking, and show that list to other providers who are treating you.

---

*PPIs: Omeprazole (*Prilosec*), esomeprazole (*Nexium*), pantoprazole (*Protonix*), lansoprazole (*Prevacid*), and rabeprazole (*Aciphex*).

such as antacids and H2-blockers,[†] also require dose separation.

- *Calcium channel blockers.*[‡] PIs and cobicistat can increase the levels of these drugs, used to treat high blood pressure, which can increase the risk of side effects.

- *Seizure medications.* It's important to check drug levels of a number of seizure medications if you're on ART to make sure you're getting the right dose. Some seizure medications can lower drug levels of some HIV drugs. Levetiracetam (*Keppra*) is a good choice if you need a seizure medication because it doesn't interact with HIV drugs.

- *Alternative therapies.* Don't forget that many **complementary medicine** and **alternative medicine** therapies, such as herbal supplements, are *drugs* from the body's point of view and can interact with prescribed medications (Questions 41 and 91).

This is *not* a complete list. When in doubt, ask your provider or pharmacist.

Complementary medicine

The use of a non-standard medical treatment in addition to standard therapy.

Alternative medicine

The use of a non-standard medical treatment in place of standard therapy.

[†]H2-blockers: Ranitidine (*Zantac*), cimetidine (*Tagamet*), and famotidine (*Pepcid*).
[‡]Calcium channel blockers: Nifedipine (*Adalat, Procardia*), verapamil (*Calan*), and diltiazem (*Cardizem, Tiazac,* and others).

PART SEVEN

Staying on Therapy

How long will therapy last?

Can therapy ever be stopped?

How will I know if my therapy stops working?

More . . .

35. How long will therapy last?

If you're taking a recommended regimen and you're not missing doses, your first regimen will last as long as you do—a lifetime! Amazingly, once you have achieved viral suppression, the virus cannot escape or form resistance. This is one of the great miracles of HIV therapy and is a big change from the bad old days when our treatments weren't sufficiently strong enough to suppress viral replication. At that time, resistance was inevitable and frequently involved **cross-resistance** to other drugs in the same class.

Cross-resistance

Resistance to one drug that results in resistance to other drugs, usually in the same class.

There might be changes in your first regimen even if the viral load remains suppressed. These would be to switch you to a better, safer, or easier to take treatment, reflecting progress in the field. The good news is that you can always go back to an older regimen if the switch doesn't work for you, as no resistance occurs provided the viral load remains undetectable.

It's theoretically possible for the benefits of a single ART regimen to be permanent as long as you continue to take it faithfully.

Therapy is said to be failing when the viral load is repeatedly greater than 200. This happens for a reason—usually someone has stopped taking the regimen regularly, or a pharmacy has made a dispensing error, or there has been some miscommunication about what to take. In such circumstances, your provider might call up your pharmacy to find out what has actually been dispensed. I can usually figure out why treatment has failed after getting this information.

Treatment interruption

Stopping antiretroviral therapy. No longer in vogue.

36. Can therapy ever be stopped?

It can, but it's always a bad idea. You should assume that once you start ART, you're in it for the long haul. We used to hear a lot about **treatment interruption (drug**

holidays or **structured treatment interuptions**). Many patients were tired of side effects and wanted a break. Researchers thought that occasional treatment interruptions—especially if done according to a schedule, or "structured"—might allow people to recover from drug toxicity without harm, provided the CD4 count stayed in a safe zone.

That approach turned out to be very wrong. A large clinical trial comparing intermittent versus continuous therapy was stopped early because people who interrupted therapy were more likely to die or have serious complications than those who remained on therapy, even if they kept their CD4 counts above 250. Not only that, when you stop therapy, the viral load will rebound (sometimes to very high levels), potentially allowing the virus to be passed onto others. In short, stopping treatment is a bad idea for multiple reasons.

That doesn't mean you can't stop treatment if you absolutely must. We sometimes have to stop therapy in people who develop serious side effects or who are too sick to take medications, or need to have surgery—but those are exceptional cases. Fortunately, now that ART has improved, staying on therapy is much easier than it used to be. In addition, if you have had long term viral suppression, it takes at least a few days before the viral load starts becoming detectable again, sometimes even a few weeks. As a result, don't panic if you must miss a day or two every now and then—just keep these misses infrequent!

Be aware that stopping NNRTI-containing regimens can be especially risky. The long half-life of drugs like efavirenz, rilpivirine, doravirine, and nevirapine means that the drugs hang around for a long time—sometimes

Drug holiday

An old term for an interruption in therapy, usually when the decision was made by the patient.

Structured treatment interruption

An old term for an interruption in therapy that was approved by the provider, generally according to a specific schedule.

STAYING ON THERAPY

You should assume that once you start therapy, you're in it for the long haul.

weeks after your last dose, and long after the other drugs in the regimen have disappeared. That's a problem, because it leaves them vulnerable to resistance when the virus starts to replicate again, and resistance to these drugs requires just a single mutation. If you should ever have to stop taking an NNRTI-based regimen, talk to your provider about safer ways to do it.

37. How will I know if my therapy stops working?

You can't tell whether therapy is working based on how you feel or what your CD4 count is. The *only* way to know is to measure the viral load, which is always the best indicator of treatment success and failure (Question 23). Your viral load should be undetectable within 4 to 6 months of starting therapy; usually this happens much faster (within 4 to 8 weeks), especially with integrase inhibitor-based regimens. If your viral load doesn't decrease the way it's supposed to, or if it becomes detectable after having been undetectable, this *may* be a sign of treatment failure.

No lab test is perfect. A viral load can be detectable in people who aren't failing, often just because lab tests aren't 100 percent accurate. If you're taking your medications faithfully and you have a viral load that's detectable but low, don't panic. It's probably just a "blip"—a single detectable viral load that generally means nothing (Question 23). The only way to tell the difference between a blip and early failure is to repeat the viral load. If its falls back to undetectable levels, then it was a blip and you should forget about it. We generally get concerned only if the viral load is repeatedly above 200.

If the viral load remains detectable above 200 or is rising, there may be a problem. This should be taken seriously—even when everything else is going great—because it could mean that you're developing resistance. We can measure resistance when the viral load is above 200. The *GenoSure Archive* test can measure resistance when the viral load is low or undetectable (Question 24).

A few people on treatment have what we call **persistent low-level viremia**. Many or most of their viral load tests have detectable virus, usually between 20 and 200 copies. Most of the time, this occurs in people who started treatment with a very high viral load and have a high viral reservoir. Changing therapy or adding drugs to the regimen (called "intensification") does not lower the viral load. While some evidence shows that persistent low-level viremia is associated with a higher risk of treatment failure, we do not find drug resistance if the viral load stays below 200 consistently, and people are taking their medications faithfully. In addition, the studies that have looked at treatment as prevention used 200 as the cut-off for what was considered "undetectable." Finally, this low level of detectable virus does not influence the CD4 cell count or lead to complications from HIV such as opportunistic infections. My advice to those with persistent low-level viremia is not to worry about the result and to continue taking their regimens regularly as recommended.

persistent low-level viremia
Viral load that is repeatedly detectable between 20 and 200 copies despite being on antiretroviral therapy.

The CD4 count is a lousy measure of treatment failure (Question 22). If your viral load is undetectable but your CD4 response is disappointing, changing medications won't make a difference. The best approach is to keep your viral load undetectable, and let the CD4 count do what it will do. In a person with an undetectable viral load, we know of no way to increase the CD4 count in a way that makes a meaningful clinical difference. That's why measuring the CD4 cell count once it is over 350 or so is now considered optional. I typically discourage my patients from checking CD4 cell counts if they have been on treatment for years, have a suppressed viral load, and have normal or near-normal results. The variation in the CD4 count at this level just causes anxiety and has no important meaning!

38. What if my virus becomes resistant to the medications?

Resistance can be the *result* of treatment failure (when you're not taking your medications properly) or it can be the *cause* of failure (when you already have resistance before you start). Resistance can occur whenever the virus is able to replicate despite the use of antiretroviral medications. Fortunately, resistance is no longer the inevitable result of ART, as it was in the bad old days. Studies show that people who take their medications faithfully rarely develop resistance.

Studies show that people who take their medications faithfully rarely develop resistance.

The best way to deal with resistance is not to let it happen. If you're about to start therapy for the first time, get a resistance test to make sure your virus is susceptible to the regimen. Once you start, take every dose, and keep your viral load suppressed. If you follow those two rules, you'll probably never have to read the rest of this answer.

The best way to deal with resistance is not to let it happen in the first place.

But, to paraphrase an oft-repeated maxim, "resistance happens." When it does, I've got two more rules: (1) Act fast. Continuing a failing regimen allows more mutations and resistance to occur. (2) Get data. Resistance testing tells you which drugs your virus is resistant to and which will still work (Question 24).

We now have a lot of drugs in different classes and with different resistance profiles. If you develop resistance on your first combination, you'll still have plenty of good options. But those options might not be quite as easy or as well tolerated as the first, so make the first one last!

39. Are new drugs being developed?

Since the approval of zidovudine (AZT, *Retrovir*) in 1987, there has been a steady increase in the number of new antiretroviral agents. The first drugs were NRTIs. Two other classes, PIs and NNRTIs, were introduced in the mid-1990s. Then came enfuvirtide (T20, *Fuzeon*), a fusion inhibitor and the first entry inhibitor. 2006 and especially 2007 were breakthrough years, with the introduction of darunavir (*Prezista*, a PI with activity against resistant virus), maraviroc (*Selzentry*), the first CCR5 antagonist; raltegravir (*Isentress*), the first INSTI; and etravirine (*Intelence*), a new "second-generation" NNRTI (Question 29). The sudden availability of multiple drugs with activity against resistant virus meant that people with HIV that had multi-class resistance could achieve viral suppression.

More breakthroughs followed: 2011 saw the approval of rilpivirine (*Edurant*), a new NNRTI, as well as *Complera*, a single-tablet regimen that contains rilpivirine, tenofovir, and emtricitabine. *Stribild*, the first single-tablet INSTI-containing regimen, was approved in 2012; the next year saw the approval of dolutegravir (*Tivicay*), followed in 2014 by *Triumeq*, another single-tablet INSTI regimen. In late 2015 and early 2016, we saw the approval of several TAF-containing combinations (*Genvoya, Odefsey, Descovy*), a further improvement over the older TDF-containing versions (*Stribild, Complera, Truvada*). In 2018, the NNRTI doravirine (*Pifeltro*) was approved, along with its single tablet regimen *Delstrigo*; that same year saw the approval of the first monoclonal antibody for HIV treatment, the attachment inhibitor ibalizumab (*Trogarzo*), the single tablet INSTI regimen Biktarvy (bictegravir/TAF/FTC), and the two-drug combination tablet for suppressed patients, *Juluca* (dolutegravir/lamivudine). Most recently, another two-drug treatment for initial therapy was approved, dolutegravir/lamivudine (*Dovato*).

The costs of bringing a new drug to market are enormous. For a drug to make it that far, it has to have a reason to exist. New drugs tend to fall into one of two categories: They either work when others don't because of a unique mechanism of action or resistance profile, or they're more convenient or less toxic than existing drugs. In addition, clinical studies must show that the drug is well absorbed, achieves adequate drug levels, suppresses viral load, and is active and safe. A lot of things can go wrong along the way, and not all drug candidates make it to the finish line.

At some point in the near future, drug companies may decide that the current therapies for HIV are good enough, that the competition is too stiff, and that there's no longer a financial incentive to develop new agents. That hasn't happened yet, but the pace of drug development has slowed, especially for drugs used to treat resistant virus, because there are so few people now with hard-to-treat virus. Don't assume there will always be new drugs to bail you out if you fail multiple regimens. Make your current regimen last by taking it as prescribed.

40. What if I decide not to take medications?

With the exception of elite controllers, all people with HIV need treatment. I sometimes hear people say they want to fight their HIV the "natural way" instead of taking "toxic chemicals." People who talk like that are sometimes too young to remember the devastation that AIDS caused during the bad years, and they're unaware of the devastation that it's still causing in parts of the world that can't afford effective therapy. They forget that "natural" doesn't necessarily mean healthy. After all, HIV is completely "natural," and it has killed millions. In contrast, those "toxic chemicals" that we doctors love to dish out have saved countless lives and represent one of the great medical miracles of the twentieth century. It's great to use "natural" approaches to treatment such as good nutrition, plenty of exercise, and attention to spiritual and mental wellness—but if you have HIV, these accompany antiretroviral therapy, they don't replace it!

Although almost everyone with HIV will benefit from ART, not everyone *needs* to be on therapy immediately. Elite controllers—people with undetectable viral loads who have normal and stable CD4 counts without ART—are the only people who may not benefit from ART (though even *that's* controversial). But elite controllers make up a tiny fraction of HIV-positive people. It is likely they control HIV because of their genetic make-up, not because of their lifestyle, diet, herbal supplements, meditation regimen, or anything else they have control over.

We've known about the devastation HIV can cause without treatment since the early 1980s. Take advantage of what medical science has to offer!

41. Should I take complementary or alternative therapies?

Complementary and **alternative medicine (CAM)** is the term used to describe non-standard therapies.

Complementary and alternative medicine (CAM)

Medical products or treatments that are not standard of care (see **Alternative medicine** and **Complementary medicine**).

Complementary medicine is the use of non-standard therapy *in addition to* standard therapy; alternative medicine is the use of non-standard therapy *instead of* standard therapy. One problem with non-standard therapies is that there usually isn't enough evidence to make them standard. That doesn't mean they don't work. Natural therapies can *become* standard. There are also examples of natural substances that are very bad for you. (Socrates didn't take hemlock for his health!)

Research into the safety and benefits of CAM *is* being conducted. In fact, the National Center for Complementary and Alternative Medicine, which is part of the **National Institutes of Health (NIH)**, now gives grants for this kind of research. In some cases, the research supports the claims made about these substances; in other cases, it doesn't. So far, there have been no alternative therapies for HIV that have come close to matching the benefits of ART.

National Institutes of Health (NIH)

An agency of the federal government (under the U.S. Department of Health and Human Services) responsible for conducting and funding medical research.

Another problem with CAM is that it often involves taking substances that can interact with ART drugs. Those who think of herbs as cuddly, benign, natural substances don't like to hear them called "drugs," but let's face it—if they weren't drugs, there would be no point in taking them. Antiretroviral medications interact with lots of other drugs, and we now know they can interact with herbal medications, too. The best studied example is St. John's wort, which lowers levels of many HIV drugs, allowing the virus to replicate and develop resistance. Unfortunately, only a few of the many CAM therapies have been tested for interactions with HIV drugs.

When I bring up the lack of research, my CAM-supporting patients and friends tell me the tests aren't done because there's no profit in it for the big bad drug companies. But, in fact, the supplement industry is making a *fortune*. It has powerful friends in Congress who fight all attempts at regulation. If they're not studying the safety or efficacy of their products, it's because they're already doing just fine without any data—just a believing public.

My advice: Follow the evidence. Be skeptical about *everything*. Whether you're thinking of taking a prescription drug or an herb, first ask, "What's the evidence that this will help me and not hurt me?" And when you're looking for that evidence, don't be like the current anti-vaxxers, HIV denialists, and "creation scientists," who define "research" as a Google search for opinions that match their own. Use credible sources, like AIDS.gov, AIDSinfo.nih.gov, and the Centers for Disease Control and Prevention website. Some additional excellent resources are included in the Appendix at the end of this book.

So far, there have been no alternative therapies for HIV that have come close to matching the benefits of ART.

42. What is immune-based therapy?

Immune-based therapy is treatment designed to restore the immune system or to improve its ability to fight HIV. It's clear that we're never going to cure HIV just by keeping the viral load undetectable with ART. The virus inserts its DNA into human cells, where it remains forever, waiting until treatment is stopped to create new virus particles. Our drugs work *only* on replicating virus; they have no activity against viral DNA that's hiding out in resting CD4 cells.

Theoretically, we could cure HIV if we could activate all resting CD4 cells and wake up the sleeping virus using "**latency**-reversing agents," allowing ART to do

Immune-based therapy
Treatment for HIV designed to affect the immune system and its response to the virus, as opposed to standard antiretroviral therapy, which suppresses the virus itself.

Latency
The ability of HIV to persist in human cells for the lifetime of an infected individual by inserting its DNA into long-lived reservoir cells.

91

Immune-based therapy is treatment designed to restore the immune system or to improve its ability to fight HIV.

Therapeutic vaccine

A vaccine given to treat an existing infection by stimulating the immune system to fight it.

its thing against the activated virus. There are two problems with this approach. First, unless you activate *every* resting CD4 cell in the body, you'll still have latent virus and be no closer to a cure than you were before. Second, resting CD4 cells aren't the only reservoirs for latent HIV, but some of the proposed treatments may activate only CD4 cells.

Another immune-based approach is therapeutic vaccination. The idea here is not to eradicate HIV but to stimulate the immune system to fight it better. A successful **therapeutic vaccine** might delay the need for ART or turn more people into elite controllers. There are vaccines being studied, but this is still an experimental approach that probably won't be put into practice any time soon.

Immune-based therapy has clearly lagged behind antiviral therapy, but that doesn't mean it doesn't have a future. However, I attended a meeting in 2002 where HIV experts were asked what they thought the next big thing would be in HIV therapy. The majority voted for immune-based therapy—and we still don't have one. Alas, they were way too optimistic! Fortunately, advances in ART have been so significant that one could argue that immune-based therapies aren't even needed.

PART EIGHT

Side Effects and Toxicity

What are the side effects of protease inhibitors?

What can I do about changes in my body shape?

How can I protect my liver?

More . . .

43. What are the side effects of protease inhibitors?

Some side effects and long-term toxicities have been attributed to PIs as a class. These include **gastrointestinal** symptoms, such as loose stools or nausea (Question 66), body shape changes (fat accumulation) (Question 46), and metabolic toxicities, such as increased levels of **cholesterol** and **triglycerides** and high blood sugar or **diabetes**. However, the recommended PI, darunavir (*Prezista, Prezcobix*), is very well tolerated and is much less likely to cause these problems than the older PIs. The same is true for atazanavir (*Reyataz, Evotaz*), an alternate PI. If any of you are on the older PIs such as indinavir (*Crixivan*), saquinavir (*Invirase*), or nelfinavir (*Viracept*), you should speak with your provider about new options that are safer.

Hyperlipidemia is an elevation of the cholesterol and/or triglyceride levels. High cholesterol can increase the risk for heart disease and stroke (Question 47). Very high triglyceride levels can cause pancreatitis. If you have high lipids on an older drug such as lopinavir/ritonavir (*Kaletra*), talk to you provider about changing to something more contemporary. You can also modify your diet, perhaps with the help of a nutritionist, and do more aerobic exercise. Depending on how bad the results are and the number of other cardiac risk factors you have, hyperlipidemia may need to be treated either with medications that lower cholesterol and/or triglycerides. The number we worry most about is the LDL ("bad") cholesterol, which we lower with statins (Question 47). Statins are being studied not only for their cholesterol-lowering effects, but also for their ability to reduce inflammation, an effect of HIV we sometimes see even in some people with viral suppression.

Gastrointestinal

Relating to the digestive tract: esophagus, stomach, small intestines, colon, and rectum.

Cholesterol

A substance found in body tissues and the blood. Cholesterol is ingested (in meat or animal products) and also manufactured by the body. Cholesterol levels are measured by blood tests.

Triglycerides

Fats that are ingested in the form of vegetable oils and animal fats.

Diabetes

A disorder resulting in elevated amounts of glucose (sugar) in the blood and urine.

Hyperlipidemia

An abnormal elevation of lipids (cholesterol and/or triglycerides) in the blood.

Insulin resistance means the body can't respond appropriately to the insulin that is produced by the **pancreas** to control blood sugar. When it's severe enough, it can lead to diabetes. We used to think of this as a PI side effect back when we were using indinavir (*Crixivan*), which no one living in the 21st century should still be taking. Insulin resistance is detected with a fasting blood sugar, hemoglobin A1C, or a glucose tolerance test. People with insulin resistance or actual diabetes need to change their diet by avoiding sugars, limiting starches, and eating small amounts throughout the day. Aerobic exercise and weight loss help a lot, but medications are often necessary, too.

Fat accumulation (or **lipohypertrophy**) is the buildup of fat in places where it doesn't belong; it is discussed further in Question 46.

Liver toxicity (or **hepatotoxicity**) can occur with any PI, but people who have chronic hepatitis B or C are at greatest risk (Question 48). Liver toxicity generally shows up in your blood test results before you feel it yourself. Tell your provider if you develop belly pain, continued nausea, loss of appetite, dark urine, or yellow skin or eyes—all are possible side effects of liver toxicity from medications.

Other PI side effects include elevation of **bilirubin** (indinavir, atazanavir), which is completely harmless but may cause jaundice (yellowing of the eyes or skin); kidney stones or kidney damage (indinavir, atazanavir); gallstones (atazanavir); dry skin, hair loss, cracked lips, and ingrown toenails (indinavir); and rash (fosamprenavir or darunavir). Again, the jaundice caused by atazanavir and indinavir is not harmful to you or your liver, but might not look good, especially in the white part of the eyes. It resolves quickly when the medications are stopped.

Insulin resistance

A condition in which the body cannot respond to insulin as well as it should. This applies both to insulin naturally produced by the pancreas and insulin injected as medication. Can lead to high blood sugar or diabetes.

Pancreas

An organ in the abdomen that makes insulin and enzymes that help digest food.

Fat accumulation (or lipohypertrophy)

A component of the "lipodystrophy syndrome" in which fat accumulates in abnormal parts of the body, such as inside the abdomen, around the neck, in the breasts, or on the upper back at the base of the neck ("buffalo hump").

Liver toxicity (or hepatotoxicity)

Damage to the liver caused by medications.

Bilirubin

A pigment produced in the liver. When bilirubin levels get too high, the skin and eyes can turn yellow ("jaundice" or "icterus"). Elevated bilirubin can be caused by hepatitis or by two antiretroviral drugs: indinavir (*Crixivan*) or atazanavir (*Reyataz*).

44. What are the side effects of non–nucleoside reverse transcriptase inhibitors (NNRTIs)?

NNRTIs have little long-term toxicity, but they do have short-term side effects you should know about:

- *Rash*. All the NNRTIs can cause a rash, usually during the first few weeks of therapy. It's an itchy, red rash, which often gets better on its own even if you continue the drug. However, severe, even life-threatening, rashes can occur, especially with nevirapine (*Viramune*). Signs of a serious rash are peeling or blistering of the skin, sores in the mouth, or fever. Nevirapine is given once a day for the first 2 weeks, and then twice a day; but never increase the dose if you have a rash. Rash can occur with efavirenz (*Sustiva, Atripla*), but it's less likely to be severe or to require stopping the drug. Rilpivirine (*Edurant, Complera, Odefsey*), etravirine (*Intelence*), and doravirine (*Pifeltro*) are less likely to cause rash, including severe rash, than either nevirapine or efavirenz.

- *Liver toxicity*. Nevirapine can cause serious, life-threatening liver toxicity during the first few weeks of therapy, especially in women who start the drug with CD4 counts above 250 or men with counts over 400. Sometimes it is accompanied by a rash and fever. Always see your provider and get blood tested before you increase the dose of nevirapine after the first 2 weeks. People with chronic hepatitis B or C can take nevirapine, but they are at higher risk for chronic liver toxicity and should be monitored carefully. Because of this side effect of nevirapine, it is rarely started today. However, if you have been taking it for years without problems, this liver toxicity will not suddenly happen to you—it's otherwise a very safe drug.

- *Hyperlipidemia.* The NNRTI efavirenz can elevate cholesterol and/or triglycerides. The other drugs in this class rarely do so.

- *Neurologic side effects.* Efavirenz often causes vivid dreams (good or bad), dizziness, and concentration difficulties during the first few days or weeks of treatment. Tips on managing these side effects are discussed in Question 52.

45. What should I know about nucleoside analog side effects?

First let's talk about the side effects of drugs from the past. These are important to know if you took them previously, as some of these side effects unfortunately are permanent. The good news is that we never use these medications anymore. If you are still receiving didanosine (ddI, *Videx*) or stavudine (d4T, *Zerit*), you should challenge your provider to find something safer for you to take; *almost* the same urgency applies to zidovudine (AZT, or ZDV, or *Retrovir*):

- *Peripheral neuropathy.* Stavudine (d4T, *Zerit*) and didanosine (ddI, *Videx*) should no longer be used. They often caused **neuropathy** (or **peripheral neuropathy**), that is, damage to the nerves in your feet and legs. The first symptoms were tingling, numbness, or burning pain in the toes. With time, it could extend up into the legs and become disabling. Unfortunately, back in the early 1990s, these were among the only options for HIV treatment we had, and the alternative was no treatment at all. As a result, some people with peripheral

Neuropathy (or peripheral neuropathy)

Damage to the nerves resulting in numbness or burning pain, usually in the feet or legs. Can be caused by HIV, some antiretroviral drugs, or other conditions.

neuropathy from these drugs had to continue them and still suffer from the symptoms today.

Lactic acidosis

A dangerous build-up of lactic acid (lactate) in the blood, which can be caused by some antiretroviral drugs and also by other medical conditions.

Hepatic steatosis ("fatty liver")

A buildup of fat in the liver that can be caused by a variety of medical conditions. When caused by antiretroviral agents, it is often accompanied by lactic acidosis.

- *Lactic acidosis and hepatic steatosis.* **Lactic acidosis** and **hepatic steatosis ("fatty liver")** are uncommon but serious side effects, mainly of stavudine, but to a lesser degree of zidovudine (AZT, *Retrovir, Combivir, Trizivir*) and didanosine. Symptoms can include shortness of breath, nausea, muscle aches, and just feeling lousy. Of course, these are common symptoms, while lactic acidosis isn't common at all. If you're having them, you probably don't have lactic acidosis, but you should still report them to your provider. Early diagnosis and an immediate change in therapy are essential because lactic acidosis can be fatal. You may see lactic acidosis listed as a side effect of the recommended NRTIs (e.g., *abacavir, tenofovir*), but that's just because they're in the same class as the drugs that *really* cause it. It is incredibly rare to get this side effect on the current recommended NRTIs.

- *Lipoatrophy.* Fat loss in the face, arms, legs, and buttocks (Question 46) can be caused by stavudine and to a lesser degree by zidovudine and possibly didanosine. Our currently recommended medications do not have this side effect.

- *Anemia.* Zidovudine can cause anemia. Symptoms include fatigue, dizziness, and shortness of breath. A standard blood test (CBC) will detect anemia.

- *Gastrointestinal side effects.* Zidovudine can cause nausea; TDF (*Viread, Truvada, Atripla, Complera, Stribild*) and TAF (*Descovy, Odefsey, Genvoya*) can also cause nausea, gas, or bloating. NRTIs generally don't cause diarrhea. Didanosine can cause pancreatitis, a dangerous inflammation of the pancreas, and non-cirrhotic portal hypertension, an often fatal liver condition that can occur years after the drug has been stopped.

- *Metabolic toxicity*. Lipid elevation and insulin resistance usually got blamed on PIs, but NRTIs can cause them, too, especially stavudine and zidovudine.

As I noted previously, none of those older drugs really should be used now, so if you're starting treatment today, you won't experience any of those serious side effects. Since even our best medications today still have some toxicity, it's important to review them now:

- *Hypersensitivity*. People taking abacavir (*Ziagen*, or part of *Epzicom*, *Trizivir*, *Kivexa*, or *Triumeq*) can develop a hypersensitivity reaction (HSR) within the first few weeks. A hypersensitivity reaction is another way of saying a severe allergic reaction. HSR feels like the flu and gets worse with each dose. Once you stop abacavir because of possible HSR, you can never take it again; there have been deaths in people who were "re-challenged" with the drug after having had HSR. Fortunately, the risk of HSR has been virtually eliminated by pre-testing for HLA B*5701. If the test is positive, consider yourself allergic and don't take abacavir in any of its forms. If you're negative, you should spend no time worrying about HSR.

- *Kidney toxicity*. Tenofovir can affect the kidneys. The risk is higher if you have kidney problems to begin with, are taking other drugs that affect kidneys, or if you're taking a protease inhibitor or the booster cobicistat. Kidney toxicity is generally gradual and is easily detected by standard blood and urine tests (Question 49). Compared to tenofovir DF (TDF), tenofovir AF (TAF) has way less kidney toxicity, which has made it easier to use than TDF, especially for people with other risk factors for kidney disease.

- *Loss of bone density.* Starting most ART regimens can cause an early loss in bone density. It's generally a small loss and doesn't continue to get worse over time, but may be a concern if you're older or already have low bone density. TDF has more of an effect on bones than other drugs, but other NRTIs (including abacavir, lamivudine, emtricitabine, and the other form of tenofovir, TAF) cause little or no loss in bone density (Question 50).

46. What can I do about changes in my body shape?

Lipodystrophy

Lipodystrophy

A general term for changes in body shape and fat distribution caused by some antiretroviral agents. Can include lipoatrophy, fat accumulation, or both.

Lipodystrophy is a term used to describe body shape changes that used to occur with older antiretroviral agents. Lipodystrophy includes **lipoatrophy** (fat loss) and fat accumulation. You can have one or the other, or—bad luck!—you can have both. Fortunately, this isn't happening with the drugs we use today, but many people still suffer from the effects of the older drugs they took in the past.

Lipoatrophy

Loss of subcutaneous fat (fat under the skin) in the legs, arms, buttocks, and face, caused by some nucleoside analog reverse transcriptase inhibitors (NRTIs).

The cause of fat accumulation is not known. It was linked to PIs, possibly because of their tendency to increase triglycerides and cause insulin resistance (Question 43), but all HIV treatments regardless of drug class can cause weight gain, and if you're not careful about diet and exercise this weight gain will be mostly fat. Some of this weight gain is a return-to-health—you're feeding yourself instead of the virus. This is particularly true if you started treatment with a very low CD4 cell count, or a very high viral load, or having a complication of having HIV. To put it simply, now that you're feeding yourself instead of the virus, you're "catching up"—gaining the weight you *would* have had if you were HIV negative and not sick from the virus.

Some recent studies have implicated integrase inhibitors as causing more weight gain than other drug classes. We do not yet know the mechanism of why this happens—is it because the integrase inhibitors are less likely to cause nausea, so people eat more? Or do they stimulate appetite in some way? Another observation is that tenofovir DF—the older form of the drug—may inhibit some ART-related weight gain, while tenofovir AF does not. As a result, people treated with TAF-based regimens have gained more weight than those taking TDF. Since TAF has overall better kidney and bone safety than TDF, my preference is still to use TAF over TDF, even with this information on weight.

This advice may sound obvious, but if you're gaining weight, you have to get off the couch, replace the potato chips with carrot sticks, and get to the gym. Diet and exercise will help, whether you've got abnormal fat accumulation or you're just plain overweight—and the benefits go beyond weight loss and include your cardiovascular and mental health. For true visceral fat accumulation, there are treatments that can help, including growth hormone (*Serostim*) and tesamoralin (*Egrifta*). They are expensive, and the fat will return after you stop taking them. Plus they really are not good options if you have diabetes or potentially even a strong family history of diabetes.

Lipoatrophy

Loss of fat in the arms, legs, and buttocks makes your veins stand out and gives you a flat or saggy butt. Loss of fat in the face gives you sunken cheeks and makes you look older or sicker than you are. Stavudine (d4T, *Zerit*) and zidovudine (AZT, *Retrovir, Combivir, Trizivir*) were the most common causes of lipoatrophy, but didanosine (ddI, *Videx*) probably caused it, too. The best way to deal with lipoatrophy is to avoid the drugs that cause it. If you wait until you've got lipoatrophy and then switch, some fat may return, but it can take a long time and may never return to normal. There are cosmetic procedures that treat lipoatrophy in the face, such as the use of "face filler" injections like polylactic acid (*Sculptra*).

Fat Accumulation

We used to see fat appear in unusual places, such as the upper back ("buffalo hump"), around the neck, in the breast tissue, or inside the abdomen. As a general rule, belly fat that you can grab between your fingers is **subcutaneous fat** (fat under the skin), which is normal and can't be blamed on your drugs. Abnormal fat is **visceral fat** (fat inside the belly), which can give you a distended, "pregnant-looking" stomach, with fat deep inside that can't be pinched.

Subcutaneous fat

Fat found under the skin.

Visceral fat

Fat present inside the abdomen, around the internal organs, rather than under the skin.

47. Am I at higher risk for heart disease?

Early studies showed that HIV-positive people are at higher risk for heart disease and heart attack than the general population. However, the increased risk was mostly due to the effects of HIV itself, and it is dramatically reduced with ART. Some antiretroviral drugs can increase the risk of heart disease, but they're mostly older drugs that we don't use anymore (Questions 43 and 47). There is an ongoing controversy about whether abacavir (*Ziagen, Epzicom, Trizivir*,

Triumeq) increases the risk of heart. Since several studies do suggest this side effect, I avoid using abacavir in patients who have any other cardiac risk factors: smoking, diabetes, high blood pressure, high cholesterol, a strong family history of heart disease, or being very inactive.

It's important to put the increased risk in context. First, your risk of a heart attack if you take ART is tiny in comparison to your risk of dying of AIDS if you don't. Second, the risk from even the older, more toxic drugs is still small in comparison to the effects of other risk factors that you have some control over, such as high cholesterol, insulin resistance and diabetes, high blood pressure, smoking, obesity, and physical inactivity. Finally, you lower your cardiac risk by treating HIV far more than you increase it by taking *any* antiretroviral drug.

Here's how to protect your heart: (1) don't smoke, (2) quit smoking, (3) *don't even think about* lighting up that cigarette, (4) get your blood pressure under control if it's high, (5) get your LDL cholesterol down if it's high, (6) keep your blood sugar in control if you've got diabetes, and (7) keep your weight down with aerobic exercise and a healthy diet. That leaves only three other risk factors—getting older, being a man (if you are one), and bad genes—and you can't do anything about them.

. . . Oh, did I mention that you shouldn't smoke?

48. How can I protect my liver?

The liver's role in our health is too complex to list completely, but it's involved in metabolism, the chemical

Detoxification

The removal of toxic substances from the body. An important function of the liver and kidneys.

reactions that take place in the cells of the body, including the **detoxification** of many of the drugs we use to treat HIV. It makes proteins, stores fuel for the body, and secretes important hormones and bile, which helps with digestion of food. Because it's so important, it's critical to keep it healthy.

Many antiretroviral drugs can hurt the liver. Almost all of the PIs can cause damage, but usually only in people who have chronic hepatitis B or C. Nevirapine (*Viramune*) can be harmful to the liver, especially in women who start ART with high CD4 counts. Stavudine (d4T, *Zerit*) and zidovudine (AZT, *Retrovir*, *Combivir*, *Trizivir*) can be harmful, too, especially if you also have lactic acidosis. Other medications commonly taken by HIV-positive people, such as cholesterol-lowering drugs, can also cause liver toxicity. Here are some tips for lowering your risk:

1. Get checked for hepatitis A, B, and C. If you're not already immune to A and B, get vaccinated (preferably *after* you've started ART and have viral suppression and an improvement in your CD4 cell count). If you have chronic hepatitis B or C, get evaluated by an expert to start treatment (Questions 79 and 80).

   In many cases, your HIV provider will also be a hepatitis expert. PCR tests are sometimes necessary to rule out hepatitis, because it's possible (though rare) to have hepatitis with negative tests.

Transaminases (or liver enzymes)

Blood tests used to look for damage to the liver.

2. Get your **transaminases** (or **liver enzymes**) checked frequently, especially when you've just started therapy. This is especially important with nevirapine (Question 44).

3. Avoid excessive alcohol use (Question 92). Don't drink at all if you have chronic hepatitis B or C.

4. Use acetaminophen, the active ingredient in *Tylenol* and many other over-the-counter remedies, in moderation; don't use it at all if you have chronic hepatitis.

5. If you're taking medications for hepatitis B, don't stop them. Stopping treatment can cause dangerous hepatitis flares.

Many people use herbal therapies, especially milk thistle, to "detoxify" or protect the liver, though it's not clear whether there's any benefit. Some "natural products" may actually hurt the liver and worsen liver disease.

49. Should I worry about my kidneys?

The kidneys are organs that filter your blood and get rid of some of the things you don't need. There are only a few things you need to know about the kidneys from an HIV standpoint.

- *HIV-associated nephropathy (HIVAN)*. For both HIV and non-HIV related diseases, black people are at much higher risk than whites and Asians when it comes to kidney problems. They're at greater risk for kidney failure due to diabetes, hypertension, and also HIV. Among HIV-positive blacks, HIVAN is a common cause of kidney failure requiring dialysis or transplantation. The first clue is that there's protein in the urine. The diagnosis is usually made by removing a small piece of the kidney with a needle (**kidney biopsy**). If you've got HIVAN, you should start ART immediately because it's the only truly

Nephropathy, HIV-associated (HIVAN)

A disease of the kidneys caused by HIV. It is seen primarily in black patients.

Kidney biopsy

A procedure in which a piece of a kidney is removed using a needle inserted through the skin in order to find out the cause of kidney disorders.

effective treatment. If there isn't already a lot of damage from HIVAN, it may be reversible. But fortunately, HIVAN will not develop when a person is on effective ART—control of the viral load means avoiding HIVAN.

- *Drug toxicity.* Indinavir (*Crixivan*), now rarely used, caused kidney stones and could damage kidney function, which are two of the many reasons we don't use it much anymore. Atazanavir (*Reyataz, Evotaz*) can do the same things, though it's far safer than indinavir. Tenofovir DF (*Viread, Atripla, Complera, Truvada, Stribild*) can also hurt the kidneys, especially in people who already have kidney problems. The newer version, tenofovir alafenamide (TAF, in *Descovy, Odefsey,* and *Genvoya*), is safer for kidneys and generally preferred. (Question 30).

- Be careful with other drugs that hurt the kidneys, such as **non-steroidal anti-inflammatory drugs (NSAIDs)** (ibuprofen, naproxen, and related drugs, which are found in many over-the-counter medications, such as *Motrin* and *Aleve*). Most NRTIs should be given at reduced doses if you have kidney problems, even though they don't directly affect the kidneys themselves. HIV-positive people often take other drugs that can cause kidney problems, including **trimethoprim-sulfamethoxazole (TMP-SMX, cotrimoxazole, *Bactrim, Septra*)**.

The kidneys are organs that filter your blood and get rid of some of the things you don't need.

Non-steroidal anti-inflammatory drugs (NSAIDs)

Drugs that are commonly used to suppress inflammation and treat pain. Some are available without a prescription.

Trimethoprim-sulfamethoxazole (TMP-SMX, cotrimoxazole, Bactrim, Septra)

An antibiotic used to treat or prevent PCP and to prevent toxoplasmosis.

Kidney problems are detected with standard monitoring tests—the serum creatinine included in the comprehensive chemistry panel and a urinalysis. These tests are done once or twice a year even in stable people on ART.

50. *Are there risks to my bones and joints?*

Bone and joint problems can be a complication of HIV, HIV therapy, or both. There are two distinct problems—osteopenia/osteoporosis and osteonecrosis:

- **Osteopenia** is loss of bone density. When it becomes severe enough, it's called **osteoporosis** (severe thinning of the bones leading to fractures). You lose some bone density after you start most ART regimens and a little more when the regimen contains tenofovir DF (TDF, *Viread*, *Truvada Atripla*, *Complera*, *Stribild*), but the amount is small, and bone density generally levels off quickly without progressing further. Tenofovir AF (TAF, *Descovy*, *Odefsey*, *Genvoya*, *BIKTARVY*) causes little or no loss in bone density. However, HIV alone causes bone loss, too, and there's evidence that people who have ever had low CD4 counts are at greater risk for bone fractures. Other risk factors for osteopenia include smoking, use of corticosteroids (prednisone), low testosterone levels (hypogonadism, Question 51), older age, and lower CD4 count. The diagnosis of osteopenia or osteoporosis is made by DEXA scan, which is now recommended as a routine test in HIV-positive men over 50 and post-menopausal women. A good diet and resistance exercise (muscle-building) can also help preserve bone density. Switching from tenofovir DF to another agent has been shown to increase bone density, and that's true if switching to the new version, tenofovir alafenamide (TAF, Question 30), or some other NRTI such as abacavir.

Osteopenia

Loss of bone density ("thinning of the bones").

Osteoporosis

Severe osteopenia, which can lead to bone fractures.

Osteonecrosis

Damage to bones at the large joints (see **Avascular necrosis**).

Avascular necrosis

Painful joint damage caused by osteone-crosis, usually affecting the hips but sometimes the shoulders.

- **Osteonecrosis** is the underlying cause of **avascular necrosis**, a destruction of large joints, usually the hips. We don't know what causes it; we only know it's more common in people with HIV. The first symptom is hip pain. Standard x-rays may not detect it; if the pain persists, and osteonecrosis is suspected, you may need an MRI of the hips to make the diagnosis. Physical therapy might help the pain, but if not, the only treatment is surgical—usually hip replacement.

51. Can HIV or ART affect my hormones?

They can. Here are some examples:

Testosterone

The male sex hormone, which can be low in some HIV-positive men.

Hypogonadism

A deficiency of testosterone, the male sex hormone.

- *Hypogonadism.* Men with HIV sometimes have low **testosterone** levels (**hypogonadism**). We see it most commonly in men with advanced HIV disease, where it's the result of being sick, but also in some healthy men on effective ART. Symptoms include fatigue, loss of interest in sex, erectile dysfunction, weight loss, muscle wasting, or the inability to gain weight. The diagnosis is made with a blood-free testosterone level, which should be drawn in the morning. The condition is treated with testosterone gels, patches, or injections. Gels and patches are preferred because they give you steadier levels and are less likely to shut off your body's own production of testosterone. Importantly, testosterone should *only* be used in men with low testosterone levels. If your levels are normal, taking testosterone will make your testicles shut down. They'll see no reason to keep producing testosterone themselves, and they'll shrivel up into tiny hazelnuts. If you didn't have hypogonadism before, you'll have it now. Also, remember that it's not *normal* for a 70-year-old retiree to have the testosterone levels of an 18-year-old high school athlete. Your goal should be to maintain levels in the lower end of the normal range, especially as you age. Older men who take excessive doses of testosterone are at greater risk for heart attack and prostate cancer.

- *Insulin resistance and diabetes.* See Question 43.

- *Thyroid disease.* Thyroid problems aren't much more common in HIV-positive people than in anyone else, but if there's any question, it's easy enough to check using a thyroid-stimulating hormone (TSH) test. On rare occasions, as the immune system improves on ART, a condition known as thyroiditis can develop, leading to excessive thyroid hormone. Symptoms of low thyroid are weight gain, hair thinning, dry skin, and fatigue. By contrast, too high thyroid can cause weight loss, diarrhea, sleep disturbance, and tremor. In severe cases the eyes may bulge out, which is proptosis.

- *Adrenal problems.* **Adrenal insufficiency** (low levels of **cortisol**, a hormone produced by the **adrenal glands**) isn't common except in people with advanced HIV disease, who may be fatigued, dizzy when they stand up, or have blood test abnormalities that are typical for this condition. **Cushing's syndrome** (excessive cortisol) and adrenal insufficiency can occur by combining PIs or cobicistat with certain steroid sprays (fluticasone, which is included in *Flonase* and *Advair*) or steroids that are injected into joints to treat pain (Question 34). If you're receiving any ART regimen with either

Adrenal insufficiency

A deficiency in the amount of cortisol produced by the adrenal gland.

Cortisol

The steroid hormone produced by the adrenal gland essential to many bodily functions, including the response to stress.

Adrenal gland

A gland in the abdomen that produces cortisol, a steroid hormone that is essential to many bodily functions, including the response to stress.

Cushing's syndrome

Excessive cortisol levels either because of overproduction by the adrenal glands or use of steroid medication.

Testosterone should only be used in men with low testosterone levels.

ritonavir or cobicistat (our two "boosters"), you should not receive these steroid treatments! Talk to your doctor about potentially safer alternatives to these steroids or, if necessary, switching the ART regimen to something that does not contain boosters.

52. Can ART affect my nervous system?

The biggest risk to your nervous system is HIV itself. Untreated HIV can lead to a number of unpleasant neurologic problems, discussed further in Question 73. To prevent these problems, take ART. HIV drugs are mostly safe when it comes to the nervous system, but there are two things you should know about—peripheral neuropathy and efavirenz side effects:

1. *Peripheral neuropathy.* Stavudine (d4T, *Zerit*) and didanosine (ddI, *Videx*) can cause pain or numbness in the feet and legs. This complication can be irreversible, which is an important reason not to be taking these drugs (Question 45).

2. *Efavirenz side effects.* People who take efavirenz (*Sustiva, Atripla*) often experience *something* abnormal with the first few doses—dizziness, vivid dreams (enjoyable or otherwise), and "brain fog" or difficulty concentrating, especially in the morning. These symptoms tend to get better with each dose and are often gone within a few days. If they last for more than 3 to 4 weeks, they probably won't get better, and you may need to change medications. Efavirenz is not as widely used in the United States as it once was, but it's still the gold standard in much of the

world. If you're taking efavirenz, here are some tips for getting used to it:

a. Take it in the evening but at least 2 hours after dinner. Taking it with fatty food can increase drug levels and side effects.

b. Don't take the first dose the night before you have something important to do. Wait until a weekend or a time when you have a few days off.

c. If you're dreaming so much that you're not getting a good night's sleep, short-term use of a **benzodiazepine** (a tranquilizer in the *Valium* class) may help suppress the dreams. (Benzodiazepines should not be used to treat *chronic insomnia*, however. They're habit-forming, and there are much better ways to treat insomnia these days.)

d. If you're too groggy in the morning, try taking it earlier in the evening.

e. Once the side effects go away, you can take it however and whenever you want, as long as you take it each day.

Rarely, efavirenz causes more severe psychiatric symptoms, such as depression or hallucinations. If you find yourself depressed or hearing voices for the first time in your life after recently starting efavirenz, change drugs *now!* If you were depressed before you started the drug, and now you're more depressed, you probably should have picked something else. Long-term effects can occur, too. If you're just "not yourself" in terms of mood or ability to think or focus, talk to your provider about whether efavirenz could be the cause. Sometimes the only

The biggest risk to your nervous system is HIV itself.

Benzodiazepine

A class of drugs used to treat anxiety and insomnia. Diazepam (*Valium*) and alprazolam (*Xanax*) are well-known examples. The drugs can be habit-forming and can interact with some antiretroviral drugs.

way to find out is to switch to a different drug and see what happens.

3. *Integrase inhibitor side effects.* INSTIs can sometimes cause nervous system side effects, though they are less common or severe than with efavirenz. Although rarely severe enough to lead to discontinuation of the drugs, insomnia and headache can occur with integrase inhibitors.

PART NINE

Opportunistic Infections and Other Complications

What are opportunistic infections?

How do I prevent or treat tuberculosis?

Can HIV cause cancer?

More . . .

Pathogen

An infectious organism (bacterium, virus, fungus, or parasite) that causes disease.

Cellular immune system

The part of the immune system most directly affected by HIV. It controls a variety of bacterial, viral, fungal, and parasitic infections.

Pneumocystis

A fungus (*Pneumocystis jiroveci*) that is a common cause of pneumonia (PCP) in people with HIV.

Cryptococcus

A fungus or yeast that is a common cause of meningitis in people with HIV.

An OI is an infection caused by an organism that is normally kept in check by the cellular immune system.

---

53. *What are opportunistic infections?*

An "opportunist" is a person who takes advantage of opportunities, usually at the expense of others, for his or her own benefit. Similarly, an opportunistic infection (OI) is one in which a **pathogen** (a bacterium, virus, fungus, or parasite) takes advantage of a weakness in the body's defense mechanisms to cause disease. In the case of HIV, an OI is an infection caused by an organism that is normally kept in check by the **cellular immune system** (the part of the immune system that is most damaged by the HIV virus*).

Some pathogens are almost exclusively opportunistic, meaning they rarely cause problems in people with normal immune systems. Examples include many of the common HIV-related OIs, such as *Pneumocystis* pneumonia (Question 54), *Cryptococcal* meningitis (Question 57), *Mycobacterium avium* **complex** (**MAC**) in the tissues and bloodstream (Question 55), and *Toxoplasma* in the brain (Question 56). Other pathogens take advantage of immunosuppressed patients but can cause disease in anyone. Examples are **herpes simplex virus HSV** (Question 89), human papillomavirus (HPV), and the bacterium that causes tuberculosis (TB) (Question 59), each of which causes more frequent or severe disease in people with low CD4 counts. In some cases, OIs can be prevented by avoiding exposure to the pathogen itself. For example, we lower the risk of spreading TB by isolating those who are actively infected; you can avoid toxoplasmosis by cooking meat properly and washing your hands carefully after changing your cat's litter box; you can avoid syphilis by wearing condoms. However, many opportunistic pathogens are ubiquitous—they're found everywhere and can't be avoided. Examples include *Pneumocystis*, MAC, and *Cryptococcus*. Prevention of infections caused by these organisms requires either prophylaxis (medical treatment that prevents disease) or better yet, ART, which keeps the CD4 count above the danger zone.

Table 5 lists most of the complications of HIV and the CD4 counts at which they occur.

*As opposed to the humoral immune system, which fights infections using antibodies.

54. What is PCP?

PCP used to stand for *Pneumocystis carinii* pneumonia, one of the most common OIs in HIV-positive patients. *Pneumocystis* started out as a parasite, but microbiologists eventually figured out it was a fungus; they also realized that the rat form of pneumocystis was "carinii," and the human form was different, so they changed the name to *Pneumocystis jiroveci*. Most people still use the abbreviation PCP, which stands for *PneumoCystis* pneumonia. Unfortunately, not everyone got the memo, so I often hear younger providers now referring to it as PJP, which sounds weird to me!

You can't avoid being exposed to *Pneumocystis*. In fact, it may live harmlessly in our lungs already, causing problems only if we become immunosuppressed. You're unlikely to get PCP if your CD4 count is above 200, or if you're on effective ART.

The most common symptoms of PCP are gradually worsening shortness of breath, chest tightness, fever, and dry cough. Many people with PCP describe that previously easy activities (walking up a flight of stairs,

Mycobacterium avium complex (MAC)

A bacterium related to tuberculosis that causes disease in people with advanced HIV disease, including fever, night sweats, weight loss, diarrhea, liver disease, abdominal pain, and anemia. Also known as *Mycobacterium avium intracellulare* (MAI).

Herpes simplex virus (HSV)

A virus that causes painful blisters and ulcers on the lips, genitals, near the anus, or on other parts of the skin.

PCP

Used to stand for *Pneumocystis carinii* pneumonia, one of the most common OIs in an HIV-positive patient. It now stands for *PneumoCystis* pneumonia, because of the change in the species name.

TABLE 5 Complications of HIV CD4 Count

CD4 count*	Infectious Complications	Noninfectious Complications
Above 500	Acute retroviral syndrome [11, 16][†] Vaginal candidiasis [75]	Persistent generalized lymphadenopathy (PGL) [11] Guillain-Barré syndrome [16] Myopathy [16] Aseptic meningitis [16]
200–500	Bacterial pneumonia [67] Pulmonary tuberculosis [59] Shingles (herpes zoster) [71] Oral candidiasis (thrush) [64] Cryptosporidiosis, acute [66, 90] Kaposi's sarcoma [61] Oral hairy leukoplakia (OHL) [64] Cervical and anal dysplasia or cancer [61, 75]	Lymphoma [61] Anemia [70] Thrombocytopenia (low platelet count) [6]
Less than 200	Pneumocystis pneumonia [54] Histoplasmosis [57] Coccidioidomycosis [57] Tuberculosis outside the lungs [59] Progressive multifocal leukoencephalopathy (PML) [72]	Weight loss and wasting [69] Peripheral neuropathy [73] HIV-associated dementia [73]
Less than 100	Toxoplasmosis [56] Cryptococcal meningitis [57] Cryptosporidiosis, chronic [66, 90] Microsporidiosis [66] Candidal esophagitis [65]	
Less than 50	CMV disease [58] MAC infection [55]	Primary central nervous system lymphoma (PCNSL) [61]

* The conditions listed can occur at CD4 counts at or below the ranges shown in this table. Most become more frequent at lower CD4 counts. While uncommon, they can also occur at CD4 counts higher than the ranges listed. These hardly ever occur in people on ART that suppresses the viral load, regardless of the CD4 cell count.
[†] Numbers in brackets refer to question numbers in this book.

Source: Adapted with permission from Bartlett, JG, Gallant JE, Pham PA. *2012 Medical Management of HIV Infection*, 16th ed. Durham, NC: Knowledge Source Solutions; 2012.

talking on the telephone) become difficult because of shortness of breath. Chest pain and yucky sputum are more typical of bacterial pneumonia, which tends to come on more suddenly.

PCP can be fatal if untreated—it was a common cause of death before we had effective treatment for HIV. Clues to the diagnosis include an abnormal chest x-ray and low oxygen levels in the blood or low measured oxygen saturation levels when your vital signs are taken. The diagnosis is made by an **induced sputum** exam, which involves inhaling a salt solution that makes you cough hard and deep, or **bronchoscopy**, where a flexible scope is used to sample fluid from your lungs. A blood test called beta glucan can also strongly suggest PCP.

It's best to confirm the diagnosis rather than just treating it based on the assumption that it's PCP, because other conditions can look just like PCP, the steroids we use to treat PCP can make other OIs worse, and side effects are common during the 3-week course of therapy.

The best treatment for PCP is trimethoprim-sulfamethoxazole (TMP-SMX, cotrimoxazole, *Bactrim*, *Septra*). There are alternatives for people who are allergic to sulfa drugs. People with moderate or severe PCP should also take prednisone, a steroid that keeps your breathing from getting worse before it gets better.

The best way to prevent PCP is to be on ART, which should keep your CD4 count well above 200. Having an undetectable viral load helps, too, regardless of your CD4 count. In fact, in a large study, no one who had an undetectable viral load with a CD4 count between 100 and 200 got PCP, even though they weren't taking prophylaxis. Still, prophylaxis is recommended if your CD4

Induced sputum

A test used to diagnose PCP or tuberculosis in which patients inhale a saline mist that makes them cough deeply. The sputum specimen is then sent to the lab for analysis. Also called "sputum induction."

Bronchoscopy

A diagnostic procedure in which a flexible tube is inserted into the lungs through the mouth (under sedation) so that samples or biopsies can be taken.

The best way to prevent PCP is to be on ART, which should keep your CD4 count well above 200.

PCP can be fatal if untreated—it was a common cause of death before we had effective treatment for HIV.

count is below 200 regardless of viral load. The best drug is low-dose TMP-SMX, but there are alternatives. If your CD4 count rises above 200 for at least 3 months, you no longer need prophylaxis. As with other OIs, PCP is much less common than it used to be thanks to effective ART.

55. What is MAC (MAI)?

MAC stands for *Mycobacterium avium* complex. It's also called MAI, for *Mycobacterium avium intracellulare*. It's a bacterium related to tuberculosis (TB), but unlike TB it rarely causes lung disease in people with HIV. (It can cause lung disease in people without HIV; that's a different problem.) For people with advanced HIV disease, MAC can cause fevers, chills, night sweats, and weight loss. It usually enters the body through the gastrointestinal or respiratory tract, then spreads to the local lymph nodes. Given enough time, MAC is disseminated, which means it's in the bloodstream and spread throughout the body. It can involve the liver (causing abnormal liver function tests), the wall of the intestines (causing wasting and diarrhea), and the lymph nodes (causing belly pain).

Colonization

The presence in the body of microorganisms (viruses, bacteria, etc.) that are not causing symptoms or disease.

Clarithromycin, azithromycin

Antibiotics that can be used to treat or prevent MAC as well as some bacterial lung infections.

Ethambutol

A drug used to treat MAC and TB in combination with other drugs.

To make a diagnosis of disseminated MAC, the organism should be grown in culture from a part of the body that's supposed to be sterile—usually the blood, but you can take cultures from bone marrow, the liver, the lymph node, or other internal organs. MAC that's found in the sputum or the stool doesn't count as disseminated infection—it may just be **colonizing** the intestines or lungs—but this can be a harbinger of disseminated disease if ART is not started soon.

Disseminated MAC requires treatment with either **clarithromycin** or **azithromycin** along with **ethambutol** and sometimes **rifabutin**. Treatment clears the blood and suppresses symptoms, but it's not a cure. MAC will return if the drugs are stopped, but if your CD4 count increases on ART to above 100 for at least 6 months, you can stop treatment.

MAC isn't a concern unless your CD4 count is below 50. We used to recommend prophylaxis for MAC for those with a CD4 cell count at this low level, but we now know that ART is much more important for preventing MAC, so we prioritize that. Like so many other OIs, you can't avoid exposure to MAC because it's everywhere. Prevention with ART or prophylaxis is the only way to prevent getting sick.

56. What is toxo?

"Toxo" is short for toxoplasmosis, a disease caused by the parasite *Toxoplasma gondii*. You get infected either by eating seriously undercooked meat (especially lamb, pork, or beef) or by exposure to cat poop (usually by accident, after not washing your hands after changing your cat's litter box). After infection, the parasite lives in your body, walled off by the immune system, and causes no harm as long as your immune system remains healthy. However, if your CD4 count falls below 100, you can get sick. The most common and serious form of toxo is **encephalitis**, in which abscesses form in the brain.

A simple blood test, the **toxoplasma antibody test** will tell you whether you carry the parasite. A positive test means that at some time in your life you were infected. Perhaps as a child you shared a sandbox with Kitty, or maybe as an adult you developed a taste for carpaccio or steak tartar. If your test is positive, keep your CD4 count

Rifabutin

A drug used to treat or prevent MAC. It is also used as an alternative to rifampin to treat tuberculosis.

Toxoplasma

A parasite (*Toxoplasma gondii*) that causes brain lesions (encephalitis) in people with HIV.

Encephalitis

An infection of the brain.

Toxoplasma antibody test

A blood test used to look for exposure to the *Toxoplasma* parasite.

MAC isn't a concern unless your CD4 count is below 50.

well above 100 with ART so your immune system can protect you. If it falls below 100, take prophylaxis, either with trimethoprim-sulfamethoxazole (TMP-SMX, co-trimoxazole, *Bactrim*, *Septra*) or with one of the alternatives to prevent encephalitis.

If you have a negative antibody test, avoid infection with the parasite, especially if your CD4 count is low. Don't eat raw or rare meat. Wear gloves in the garden, and wash your hands after digging in the dirt. Get someone else to change the litter box for you or use the appropriate precautions. There's no need to trade Kitty in for Fido if you're careful (Question 94). Studies show no increased risk of toxo in cat owners.

Toxoplasmic encephalitis (also called "CNS toxo") starts out with headache and/or neurologic symptoms such as seizures or weakness affecting one side of the body. It's treatable, but only with a combination of several unpleasant medications taken at high doses for at least 6 weeks, followed by lower doses until your CD4 count goes up with ART. Prevention is definitely the way to go.

Cryptococcal meningitis

Meningitis (infection of the spinal fluid and spinal cord lining) caused by *Cryptococcus*.

Meningitis

An infection or inflammation of the spinal fluid and the lining of the spinal cord.

57. What about cryptococcal meningitis and other fungal infections?

Cryptococcal meningitis is an infection of the spinal fluid and lining of the brain with *Cryptococcus*, a yeast (fungus) that is found in the soil and inhaled into the lungs. Although people infected with *Cryptococcus* can develop pneumonia, skin lesions, or other symptoms, most develop **meningitis**, with gradually worsening headache and fever. Unlike bacterial meningitis, which makes you very sick very fast, crypto comes on more gradually. However, if left untreated, it can lead to blindness, deafness, and death. It's unlikely to occur in people with CD4 counts above 100.

A simple blood test, the serum **cryptococcal antigen** (CRAG), is almost always positive in people with cryptococcal meningitis. If it's positive, you need an immediate **spinal tap** (or **lumbar puncture**) to confirm the diagnosis and to help determine the severity. Treatment usually involves at least 2 weeks of **amphotericin B** given by vein, often with **flucytosine (5-FC)**, followed by a long course of **fluconazole**, given by mouth. In severe cases, frequent spinal taps may be needed to lower the spinal fluid pressure during the first few days of therapy. When people die of crypto, it's either because they waited too long to get treated or because they had high spinal fluid pressure that wasn't treated aggressively enough.

Once you've been diagnosed with cryptococcal meningitis, you need to stay on fluconazole to prevent **relapse** until your CD4 count has increased with ART (above 200 for at least 6 months). There's no clear way to prevent initial infection with *Cryptococcus* because it's such a common organism.

While we're on the subject of serious fungal infections, it's worth mentioning a few more. **Candidiasis** is discussed in Questions 64, 65, and 75. **Histoplasmosis** is caused by *Histoplasma capsulatum,* a fungus that's common in the Ohio and Mississippi River Valleys. **Coccidioidomycosis ("valley fever")** is caused by *Coccidioides immitis,* a fungus found in the valleys and deserts of the Southwestern United States and northern Mexico. Both can cause lung disease in people with normal immune systems, but they can cause more severe,

Cryptococcal antigen

A lab test performed on either blood or spinal fluid used to diagnose cryptococcal meningitis.

Spinal tap (or lumbar puncture)

A procedure in which a needle is inserted into the back between the vertebrae to collect a sample of cerebrospinal fluid (CSF) to diagnose meningitis.

Amphotericin B

An intravenous drug used to treat serious fungal infections.

Flucytosine (5-FC)

A drug used to treat fungal infections, usually in combination with amphotericin.

Fluconazole

A drug used to treat fungal infections.

Relapse

The return of an illness or disease, usually in someone with a chronic condition.

Candidiasis

An infection caused by *Candida,* a common yeast.

OPPORTUNISTIC INFECTIONS

Histoplasmosis

A disease caused by *Histoplasma capsulatum*, a fungus found mostly in the Ohio and Mississippi River Valleys, which causes lung infection in people with normal immune systems, and infection of the lungs and other organs in people with low CD4 counts.

widespread disease, including meningitis, in people with low CD4 counts. You can get infected by inhaling contaminated dust, and the fungus can live in your body and wait until your CD4 count is low to cause disease. If you're immunosuppressed (particularly before starting ART), and you've been living or vacationing in the Midwest or Southwest, it's worth mentioning this to your providers, in particular if you start having any unexplained symptoms.

58. What is CMV?

Coccidioidomycosis ("valley fever")

A disease cause by *Coccidioides immitis*, a fungus found mostly in the deserts and valleys of the southwestern United States and northern Mexico. It can cause lung disease, meningitis, and infection of other organs.

Cytomegalovirus (CMV) means "big cell virus," because cells infected with CMV are large. CMV is a type of **herpesvirus**, and like all herpesviruses, you can't get rid of it once you've got it. Because it's common and easily transmitted sexually, most people with HIV have already been infected.

CMV is rarely a problem for people with normal immune systems, including HIV-positive people with even moderate CD4 counts. You don't have to worry about CMV if your CD4 count is above 50, or if you're on effective ART. The most common complication of CMV is **retinitis**, an infection of the retina (the back of the eye), which can lead to blindness if not treated. See an ophthalmologist regularly, and report visual changes to your doctor *immediately* if you have a low CD4 count.

Cytomegalovirus (CMV)

A virus that can infect the eyes, the gastrointestinal tract, the liver, and the nervous system in people with advanced HIV. The most common cause of retinitis (infection of the back of the eye).

CMV can also cause gastrointestinal problems, including painful ulcers in the esophagus (**esophagitis**) (Question 64), or infection of the stomach (**gastritis**), small intestines (**enteritis**), or colon (**colitis**), causing diarrhea and abdominal pain. CMV can also affect the nervous system, causing infection of the brain (encephalitis), the spinal cord (**myelitis**), or the spinal nerves (**radiculitis, radiculopathy**).

A positive **anti-CMV IgG antibody test** means you've got the virus. Most HIV-positive people are positive, and there's not much to do about it other than to keep your CD4 count high. If the test is negative, avoid CMV infection: Practice safe sex, and if you should ever need a transfusion, it should be with CMV-negative blood.

59. How do I prevent or treat tuberculosis?

Anyone can get tuberculosis (TB), but the risk is higher for people with HIV, increasing as the CD4 count falls. People with low CD4 counts can get more severe TB, which can spread throughout the body, involving organs other than the lungs. You become infected with *Mycobacterium tuberculosis* (the TB bacterium) through close contact with someone who has active TB and is coughing. Infection doesn't always lead to illness. Your body may be able to control the organism on its own, especially if you have a high CD4 count. But if the CD4 count falls, your immune system may no longer be able to protect you.

Everyone with HIV should be tested for TB infection either with a tuberculin skin test (TST, also known as a PPD) or an interferon-gamma release assay (IGRA) blood test such as *QuantiFERON-TB Gold* or T-SPOT.TB. A positive test doesn't mean you have active TB, but it does mean you've been exposed to the organism and that it's lying dormant in your body (latent tuberculosis infection, or LTBI). If you

Herpesvirus

A family of viruses that can cause acute infection but that also remain latent in the body and recur. Examples of herpesviruses include herpes simplex virus (HSV-1 and HSV-2), varicella-zoster virus (VZV), cytomegalovirus (CMV), Epstein-Barr virus (EBV), and human herpesvirus-8 (HHV-8).

Retinitis

An infection of the retina (the interior surface of the back of the eye), which can lead to blindness if not treated. Most often caused by CMV.

Esophagitis

Infection or inflammation of the esophagus.

Gastritis

Infection or inflammation of the stomach.

Enteritis

Infection or inflammation of the small intestines.

Colitis

Infection or inflammation of the colon (large intestine).

Myelitis

Infection or inflammation of the spinal cord.

Radiculitis (radiculopathy)

Infection or inflammation of the nerves that emerge from the spinal cord.

Anti-CMV IgG antibody test

A blood test used to look for infection with CMV.

Isoniazid (INH)

A drug used to treat or prevent tuberculosis.

Anyone can get tuberculosis (TB), but the risk is much higher for people with HIV.

have LTBI based on a positive test, if you've been in close contact with someone with active TB, or if there's evidence of old TB on your chest x-ray, we generally use a 9-month course of **isoniazid** (**INH**) to kill the bacteria and prevent TB. Most shorter regimens are not yet recommended for people with HIV, but rifampin for 4 months is a good alternative. (Be careful—rifampin interacts with many medications, including ART.) TB tests are less accurate if you're immunosuppressed, so they should be repeated after your CD4 count has increased on ART.

Symptoms of active TB include prolonged fever, night sweats, weight loss, and cough with yucky or bloody sputum; other symptoms depend on the parts of the body involved. The diagnosis is usually made with sputum tests, though bronchoscopy or biopsies of the affected organs may sometimes be necessary. TB is curable with a 6-month course of therapy involving a combination of drugs. Because it's so contagious, treatment may be managed in conjunction with the health department, using **directly observed therapy** (**DOT**).

60. How do I prevent opportunistic infections?

Prophylaxis is a fancy term for prevention. When we talk about prophylaxis, we're referring to the use of a drug to prevent an opportunistic infection (OI). If your viral load is undetectable and your CD4 count is high, you don't need to worry, but if your CD4 count is low, here's what you should do to prevent some OIs:

- *PCP.* Start prophylaxis with trimethoprim-sulfamethoxazole (TMP-SMX, cotrimoxazole, *Bactrim*, *Septra*) when your CD4 count is less than

200. If you can't take TMP-SMX use **dapsone,** aerosolized **pentamidine,** or **atovaquone** (*Mepron*) (Question 54).

- *Toxoplasmosis.* Start prophylaxis if you have a positive anti-*Toxoplasma* IgG antibody *and* your CD4 count is less than 100. If you're already taking TMP-SMX, you're covered (but make sure you're taking a double-strength tablet daily). If you can't take TMP-SMX, use a combination of dapsone, **pyrimethamine,** and **leucovorin** (or **folinic acid**). If your antibody is negative, avoid exposure (Questions 56 and 94).

- *Mycobacterium avium complex* (*MAC*). Prophylaxis isn't recommended anymore. The best way to prevent MAC (and all OIs) is to go on ART (Question 55).

- *Cytomegalovirus* (*CMV*). Prophylaxis isn't recommended. Most people with HIV have already been exposed and are at risk for getting sick only if their CD4 count falls below 50 (Question 58).

- *Fungal infections* (Candida and *cryptococcal meningitis*). Unless you've already had one of these infections, prophylaxis isn't recommended (Question 57).

- *Herpes and shingles.* If you've never had these problems, prevention is not recommended. If you have frequent bouts of herpes (several per year), consider chronic suppression with **acyclovir, valacyclovir,** or **famciclovir.** Shingles rarely strikes more than once, but when it does, prophylaxis is sometimes necessary (Question 60). There's a new shingles vaccine that is recommended for all people over 50, including people with HIV who are on ART.

Directly observed therapy (DOT)

A program in which treatment is given to a patient directly by a healthcare professional, at home or in a clinic, in order to ensure that it's taken. Most common with treatment for tuberculosis but sometimes used for HIV therapy.

Dapsone

A drug used to treat or prevent PCP and to prevent toxoplasmosis.

Pentamidine

A drug used to treat PCP. Aerosolized pentamidine is sometimes used as an inhaled mist to prevent PCP.

Atovaquone (*Mepron*)

A drug used to treat or prevent PCP.

Pyrimethamine

A drug used to treat or prevent PCP or toxoplasmosis.

Leucovorin (or folinic acid)

A drug used to prevent bone marrow toxicity due to pyrimethamine.

Acyclovir

A drug used to treat herpes simplex and varicella-zoster virus.

Valacyclovir

A drug used to treat herpes simplex and varicella-zoster virus.

Famciclovir

A drug used to treat herpes simplex and varicella-zoster virus.

Kaposi's sarcoma (KS)

A tumor caused by a virus that is more common in people with HIV, especially gay men. Although it usually affects the skin, KS can also affect other parts of the body, including the gastrointestinal tract and lungs.

Human herpesvirus-8 (HHV-8)

The virus that causes Kaposi's sarcoma, Castleman's syndrome, and some rare lymphomas. Also called Kaposi's sarcoma–associated herpesvirus (KSHV).

61. Can HIV cause cancer?

People with HIV are at increased risk for certain cancers, though they're far less common than OIs. The cancers most strongly associated with HIV are discussed here:

- **Kaposi's sarcoma** (**KS**) was a huge problem during the early years of the epidemic; fortunately, we see very little of it now in the United States. (It remains a common HIV-related problem in parts of the world, in particular Africa.) It's caused by a virus, **human herpesvirus-8** (**HHV-8**), also known as **Kaposi's sarcoma–associated herpesvirus** (**KSHV**). For reasons that aren't completely understood, KS occurs mostly in gay and bisexual men. It typically causes raised, purple-colored skin lesions, but it can also affect the mouth, lungs, gastrointestinal tract, and other organs. Mild cases can be treated with topical therapies applied to the skin lesions themselves, but more severe cases need to be treated with cancer chemotherapy. Although it often gets better with HIV therapy, KS can sometimes occur even with high CD4 counts.

- Lymphoma doesn't happen often, but it's a serious problem when it occurs. The most common type is **non-Hodgkin's lymphoma** (**NHL**), but people with HIV also have an increased risk of **Hodgkin's disease** and **Burkitt's lymphoma**. Lymphoma can pop up just about anywhere in the body and is diagnosed by taking a piece of abnormal tissue (**biopsy**). It responds well to chemotherapy, but the outcome depends on the CD4 count. Being on effective ART can make a big difference in reducing the risk of lymphoma.

- **Primary central nervous system lymphoma (PCNSL)**, a lymphoma of the brain, is the cancer you'd *least* want to have. Fortunately, it almost never happens in people with CD4 counts above 50. It's treated with radiation, but in the bad old days, the prognosis was miserable. Things are a little better now—still, this is a dreaded complication of advanced HIV disease, to be avoided by taking ART.

- **Cervical cancer** and **anal cancer** are caused by human papillomavirus (HPV), a sexually transmitted virus that causes dysplasia (abnormal cells), which can eventually turn into cancer if not treated. Women should get regular Pap smears to diagnose dysplasia and prevent cancer. Anal Pap smears are now being done, too, especially in women and gay and bisexual men (Question 81). Everyone under 27 should receive the HPV vaccine to help prevent these cancers (Question 26); you can also discuss with your provider getting the HPV vaccine up to the age of 45. I would recommend it!

I've discussed the most common HIV-related cancers, but it's possible that HIV-positive people may be at higher risk for some other cancers as well, in particular lung cancer, another great reason not to smoke! Being on ART probably helps; starting it early may help even more. Make sure you're up to date on standard age-based cancer screening tests (colonoscopy, mammogram, prostate-specific antigen [PSA], etc.).

62. What is immune reconstitution?

Immune reconstitution refers to the repair of the immune system with ART. That's usually a good thing,

Kaposi's sarcoma–associated herpesvirus (KSHV)

An alternative name for human herpesvirus-8 (HHV-8), which causes Kaposi's sarcoma.

Non-Hodgkin's lymphoma (NHL)

The most common type of lymphoma in people with HIV.

Hodgkin's disease

A type of lymphoma that is more common in people with HIV but is less common than non-Hodgkin's lymphoma (NHL).

Burkitt's lymphoma

A type of lymphoma that is seen more frequently in people with HIV common than non-Hodgkin's lymphoma (NHL).

Cervical cancer and anal cancer are caused by human papillomavirus (HPV), a sexually transmitted virus that causes dysplasia (abnormal cells).

Biopsy

A procedure in which a piece of tissue is removed, either with a needle through the skin, through a scope placed in the lungs or gastrointestinal tract, or by a surgical procedure. The specimen is then examined under a microscope and/or submitted for culture to make a diagnosis.

Primary central nervous system lymphoma (PCNSL)

A lymphoma involving the brain, seen only in people with advanced HIV disease.

Cervical cancer

Cancer of the cervix (the mouth of the uterus) caused by HPV.

except when it leads to the **immune reconstitution inflammatory syndrome** (**IRIS**). IRIS occurs when body's newly restored ability to fight infections creates problems.

Let's use MAC as an example (Question 55). You don't get MAC unless your immune system is severely damaged, usually with a CD4 count below 50. At that point, your immune system is incapable of fighting off the MAC bacteria that are running rampant in the body. However, if you start ART when you have MAC, your immune system may recover enough to start doing its job. It will form walls around the bacteria, leading to abscesses or enlarged, inflamed lymph nodes. The immune response may cause fever, night sweats, and weight loss.

IRIS can occur with a variety of organisms. The most common are MAC and TB, but it can also happen with CMV, *Pneumocystis*, *Cryptococcus*, and others. People sometimes have outbreaks of shingles or herpes after they start ART. Even Kaposi's sarcoma and **progressive multifocal leukoencephalopathy** (**PML**), which usually get better with ART, can sometimes get worse.

As unpleasant as IRIS can be, it's temporary and a sign that your immune system is recovering. In almost all cases, you should continue ART! Untreated HIV is much worse than IRIS. It's important to diagnose the underlying OI, usually with a biopsy, and then treat it. Steroids (prednisone) are sometimes used to help get people through IRIS by blunting the immune response to the organism while still allowing ART to suppress HIV. The prednisone dose can be gradually lowered until the symptoms are gone.

63. *Will HIV or ART make me age faster?*

There's been a lot of talk recently about "accelerated aging" with HIV. The term is scary and a little misleading. It doesn't mean you'll get gray hair and wrinkles sooner, or that the overall aging process is being sped up, or that you're on a faster pace to the grave. Instead, it refers to the fact that some of the complications of aging are being seen more often or at younger ages in some HIV-positive people. Examples include heart disease, osteoporosis, cancer, and changes in brain function, including dementia.

There are many unanswered questions about HIV and aging, which is now the subject of a great deal of speculation as well as scientific research:

1. *Is "premature aging" caused by HIV, ART, or both?* HIV itself is mostly to blame. People who start ART with low CD4 counts are at greater risk for heart disease, bone fractures, and cognitive impairment (brain disease). People who spend a lot of time with high viral loads are at greater risk of lymphoma and other complications. ART goes a long way toward preventing the long-term complications of HIV, but ART isn't completely off the hook, because treatment with some drugs may increase the risk of kidney disease, loss of bone density, and heart disease. We do know that ART does a lot more good than harm. And today's ART is much safer than the treatments we used in the early days of HIV therapy.

2. *How does HIV accelerate aging?* Inflammation and immune activation that occur with

Anal cancer

Cancer of the anus caused by HPV.

Immune reconstitution inflammatory syndrome (IRIS)

A condition that sometimes occurs in people with low CD4 counts who start ART in which the improved immune system reacts to organisms (such as MAC, the TB bacterium, or fungi), causing illness, including fevers, weight loss, swollen lymph nodes, or abscesses.

Progressive multifocal leukoencephalopathy (PML)

A viral infection of the brain caused by JC virus, which results in progressive neurologic deterioration.

HIV are probably responsible (Question 9). These are the most likely reasons for the increased risk of aging complications. ART dramatically reduces these processes, which explains many of its long-term benefits.

3. *Can HIV cause premature aging despite effective ART?* ART clearly slows this process, but we don't know whether starting ART early, at a high CD4 count, will completely eliminate the long-term risks. (I suspect it will.) People on ART have much lower levels of inflammation and immune activation than people who aren't being treated, but their levels may still be slightly higher than in HIV-negative people. We'll need more time to find out whether someone with optimally treated HIV can expect the same quality of life as someone without HIV.

For now, the best way to stay healthy into your old age is to keep your viral load suppressed on ART, to be taking the safest possible HIV medications, and then to follow all the same many recommendations we give to people without HIV so that we can lead long, healthy lives. And if you want to stop one proven cause of premature aging, quit smoking!

PART TEN

Symptoms

What can I do about nausea and diarrhea?

What if I get a cold or the flu?

Why am I tired?

More . . .

Oropharyngeal candidiasis

Candida (yeast) infection involving the mouth and throat, including thrush, angular cheilitis, and erythematous candidiasis.

Candida

A fungus (yeast) that can cause thrush, esophagitis, and vaginitis in people with HIV.

Oral hairy leukoplakia (OHL)

Painless white plaques, or "stripes," on the sides of the tongue caused by Epstein-Barr virus.

Epstein-Barr virus (EBV)

A herpesvirus that causes infectious mononucleosis ("mono"), oral hairy leukoplakia, and some lymphomas.

Erythematous candidiasis

An infection of the mouth caused by *Candida* in which the roof of the mouth (palate) becomes red and sometimes painful.

64. What's wrong with my mouth?

The most common cause of mouth and throat problems in people not on ART is **oropharyngeal candidiasis** ("thrush"), a buildup of *Candida* (a common yeast or fungus). Thrush is easy to diagnose with a mirror and a flashlight. You'll see whitish-yellow, curd-like patches, especially on the roof and sides of the mouth, the back of the throat, and the gums. These patches can be easily scraped off. Don't confuse a white coating on the tongue with thrush. The tongue is usually the last part of the mouth to be infected, and a white coating on the tongue, with no other evidence of thrush, is usually just . . . a white coating on the tongue. Oral surgeons and dentists will tell you that there is a lot of variability in what a normal tongue can look like!

Thrush can also be confused with **oral hairy leukoplakia (OHL)**, a condition caused by **Epstein-Barr virus (EBV)** that looks like a white racing stripe down both sides of the tongue. Unlike thrush, it can't be scraped off. *Candida* can cause other mouth problems besides thrush—**erythematous candidiasis** (redness on the roof of the mouth that is sometimes painful) and **angular cheilitis** (cracks at the corners of the lips).

Painful ulcers in the mouth can be caused by viruses, but they're more often **aphthous ulcers**, more commonly known to the non-medical public as canker sores. "Aphthous," in addition to being a good word for a spelling bee, essentially means that we have no idea what causes them. The diagnosis of most of these conditions is usually based on appearance alone; special tests aren't necessary. On rare occasions, a biopsy might be done by an oral surgeon.

Thrush and OHL are fairly benign conditions, but they both indicate that something's seriously wrong with your immune system and that you should have started ART earlier. Thrush is treated with antifungal medication: either oral fluconazole or medications that treat only the surfaces, such as **clotrimazole troches** (lozenges) or **nystatin** mouth rinses. Because it's harmless, we don't usually treat OHL except with ART—it usually resolves after people have been on treatment for a few months.

Before we leave the mouth, don't forget your teeth and gums. People with low CD4 counts are at risk for serious mouth infections. Brushing, flossing, and seeing a dentist and oral hygienist on a regular basis are important to keep your teeth and gums in good shape.

65. Why does it hurt to swallow?

There are two medical terms for swallowing symptoms—**dysphagia** (difficulty swallowing) and **odynophagia** (painful swallowing), but the distinction is less important than the location. Is the problem confined to the back of the throat (**pharynx**) or does it extend into the chest (**esophagus**)? For mouth and throat symptoms, see Question 64.

When the problem is in the chest, it can be a sign of esophagitis, an inflammation of the esophagus, the tube that connects your throat with your stomach. The most common cause is *Candida,* the same yeast (fungus) that causes thrush and **vaginitis**. People with *Candida* esophagitis usually have a CD4 count below 100. Since *Candida* is the most common cause of esophagitis, the usual approach is to treat with fluconazole and see what

Thrush and OHL are fairly benign conditions, but they both indicate that something's seriously wrong with your immune system.

Angular cheilitis

Cracking of the corners of the lips, sometimes caused by *Candida*.

Aphthous ulcers

Painful ulcers in the mouth (aphthous stomatitis) or esophagus (aphthous esophagitis) that can occur in people with HIV. Called "canker sores" by non-medical people. The cause is unknown.

Clotrimazole troches

Antifungal lozenges used to treat thrush.

Nystatin

An antifungal mouth rinse used to treat thrush.

Dysphagia
Difficulty swallowing.

Odynophagia
Painful swallowing.

Pharynx
Throat.

Esophagus
The tube that connects the mouth and throat to the stomach.

Vaginitis
Infection or inflammation of the vagina.

Endoscopy
A medical procedure in which a flexible tube is inserted into the esophagus and stomach through the mouth, while the patient is sedated, in order to take samples or biopsies or to treat a variety of conditions.

happens. If *Candida* is the cause, you'll be swallowing easier within a day or two, often after just one dose. If not, you'll need an **endoscopy**, an outpatient procedure in which a flexible tube with a camera is passed from the mouth into the esophagus so that pictures and biopsies can be taken.

Other causes of esophagitis are herpes simplex virus (HSV), cytomegalovirus (CMV), and aphthous ulcers, each of which causes painful ulcers in the wall of the esophagus. The treatment of these conditions depends on the cause. Drug-resistant *Candida* can also cause esophagitis and must be treated with other antifungal drugs. It is very rare to see these problems among people with HIV who are taking ART and have viral suppression.

Of course, HIV-positive people can also develop the same esophageal problems that HIV-negative people get, including esophageal reflux, spasm, cancer, or strictures. Pills can get stuck on the way down and irritate the esophagus, so always take your meds with plenty of water.

66. What can I do about nausea and diarrhea?

In people with HIV, nausea can be caused by medications. Zidovudine (AZT, *Retrovir, Combivir, Trizivir*) and some of the older protease inhibitors were the most common offenders. If your nausea began as soon as you started a new drug, then there's no mystery about the cause. In some cases, the nausea may improve with time or by taking the pills with food. Your doctor can also prescribe medications for nausea, but if the problem persists, you may have to change drugs, and that would be the first thing I'd suggest for someone taking an outdated drug like AZT. If you've developed nausea but haven't recently changed or added medications, then it's important to look further for a cause.

Diarrhea can be caused by medications, too, especially some of the older PIs. The best way to treat drug-related diarrhea—aside from switching drugs—is with daily fiber supplements, such as psyllium. Don't be put off by the word "laxative" on the bottle. Fiber supplements add bulk to the stool, which is a good thing whether you've got diarrhea or constipation. If they don't work, ask your doctor about prescribed or over-the-counter anti-diarrhea medications or about making a change in your regimen. In rare cases of ongoing diarrhea with no identified cause, a medication called crofelemer might help.

There are many infectious causes of diarrhea, including common viruses, bacteria, and parasites. Some of these organisms, such as *Cryptosporidium*, **microsporidia**, *Isospora belli* (which causes **isosporiasis**), and *Salmonella*, are opportunistic—they occur or are more severe because of immunosuppression. Advanced HIV itself can also cause diarrhea. If you have prolonged diarrhea that isn't caused by medications, you'll need to be evaluated: first with stool studies, and if those are negative, with a scope (flexible tube with a camera), either from above (endoscopy), from below (**colonoscopy**), or both.

Diarrhea caused by viruses or food poisoning usually gets better on its own after a few days, but get medical attention if you have persistent diarrhea, or if you have fever, belly pain, blood in your stool, dizziness, or weight loss that doesn't get better even after the diarrhea

Cryptosporidium

The parasite that causes cryptosporidiosis, which can cause chronic diarrhea in immunosuppressed people. The organism can be found in contaminated water or transmitted from person to person.

Microsporidia

A variety of opportunistic parasites that cause chronic diarrhea in people with low CD4 counts.

Isosporiasis

A disease caused by the parasite *Isospora belli*, which causes chronic diarrhea in people with low CD4 counts. Uncommon in the United States and other developed countries.

Salmonella

A group of bacteria that can cause severe diarrhea, fever, and bloodstream infections. Can be transmitted through eating inadequately cooked food, especially eggs, chicken, and other meat.

Candida *is the most common cause of esophagitis.*

Colonoscopy

A medical procedure in which a flexible scope is inserted into the rectum and colon through the anus, while the patient is sedated, in order to look for abnormalities and take biopsies.

improves. When you have diarrhea, eat a bland diet with no milk products, and hydrate, hydrate, hydrate!

67. What do I do about cough or shortness of breath?

The possible causes of cough or shortness of breath depend on your CD4 count. If it's well above 200, then the list is essentially the same as it would be in an HIV-negative person. Cough can be due to the common cold, bronchitis, pneumonia, asthma, smoking, the use of certain medications, or esophageal reflux (stomach acid going up into the esophagus instead of staying in the stomach). Shortness of breath can be due to asthma, pneumonia, anemia, or acidosis (a buildup of acid in your blood). The kind of cough you get with a common cold or bronchitis doesn't usually require medical attention (Question 68). If you recently had a cold and now have one of those nagging, hacking coughs that gets worse when you laugh, exercise, or go out in the cold, you may have **bronchospasm** (or **reactive airways**), which can be treated with an inhaled bronchodilator such as albuterol.

Bronchospasm (or reactive airways)

The tendency of the bronchi (airways in the lung) to constrict (narrow), causing shortness of breath or cough. This can be chronic (in patients with asthma, for example) or temporary, following an upper respiratory infection.

The same is true if your CD4 count is low, except that now there's a longer list of possible causes. If your count is below 200, you may have PCP. With a count less than 100, there's a risk for pneumonia caused by *Cryptococcus*, *Toxoplasma*, or *Histoplasma*, which are less common than PCP (Question 54). HIV-positive people are at much higher risk for TB at any CD4 count, and the risk gets higher as the CD4 gets lower (Question 59).

You should get medical attention if you have a severe cough or one that doesn't get better with time or if you have a high fever, chest pain when you take a deep breath, shortness of breath, or are coughing up blood. You should never ignore shortness of breath or any change in your ability to exert yourself. If you're winded after climbing one flight of stairs but could climb three flights a month ago, you need to get checked out.

68. What if I get a cold or the flu?

HIV-positive people get colds and flu just like everyone else. The symptoms and duration of the illness are the same, and they're at no greater risk from complications. That's because viruses that cause the cold and flu are controlled by the **humoral (antibody-mediated) immune system,** not the cellular immune system that uses CD4 cells and is damaged by HIV.

For that reason, you don't need to do anything special if you get a cold—just rest, drink fluids, and take whatever over-the-counter cold remedy will treat the symptoms you're experiencing. These medications don't interact with HIV drugs, and you're unlikely to get anything better by prescription.

You don't need antibiotics! Your illness is caused by a virus; antibiotics kill only bacteria. They're often prescribed to keep patients happy and coming back, which is contributing to a huge drug resistance problem worldwide. This applies to **bronchitis** and most forms of **sinusitis** and sore throat as well. Studies have shown that antibiotics are no better than placebo to treat bronchitis. Cough medicine and sometimes an inhaled bronchodilator may help you feel better, but as with the common cold, you just have to ride it out—in studies of uncomplicated cough illness after colds, a significant fraction of people are still highly symptomatic 10 to 14 days

You should never ignore shortness of breath or any change in your ability to exert yourself.

Humoral (antibody-mediated) immune system

The part of the immune system that uses antibodies to fight infection. It is less affected by HIV than the cellular immune system.

Bronchitis

An infection of the bronchi (airways), usually caused by a viral infection and often occurring after a common cold.

Sinusitis

An infection of the sinuses, which are air spaces in the head connected to the nasal passages.

after the study started. It's frustrating, but be reassured that provided you are not having other worrisome symptoms (fever, shortness of breath, weight loss), you will eventually get better—even if it's never fast enough!

Sore throats require antibiotics only if they're caused by group A strep (**strep throat**) or gonorrhea, but otherwise they're likely to be viral and should be treated with throat lozenges. Most people with colds will have sinus congestion at some point. Sinusitis should only be treated with antibiotics if it's severe or prolonged. When an adult has ear pain during a cold, it's rarely an ear infection, but usually just congestion of the eustachian tubes, treated with decongestants. If we want to have antibiotics around to treat serious bacterial infections, we need to stop using them to treat viral infections that get better just as fast on their own.

Strep throat

The common term for *streptococcal pharyngitis,* a bacterial infection of the throat caused by group A beta-hemolytic *Streptococcus.*

The one infection we *do* want to treat with antibiotics is **pneumonia**, which will usually give you some combination of fever, cough, chest pain, and/or shortness of breath. It will feel much worse than the common cold or bronchitis. There is *no* evidence to support the use of antibiotics to prevent a cold from "going into the chest" or "preventing pneumonia." They're completely different diseases.

Pneumonia

An infection of the air spaces of the lungs, which can be caused by a variety of infectious organisms.

Get a flu shot every fall. If you develop true influenza during flu season, the use of anti-influenza drugs can shorten the course of the illness a little, but only if used within the first few days.

69. Why am I losing weight?

During the dark days before effective ART, weight loss was almost universal as AIDS progressed, and many patients experienced terrible wasting before they died. Weight loss is uncommon now that we have effective therapy for HIV and it's usually caused by something else. Here are some common, treatable causes of weight loss:

1. *Untreated HIV.* If you're losing weight because of HIV you need to be on ART. Weight loss is more likely to occur if you have a high viral load or a low CD4 cell count.

2. *Hypogonadism.* Men with low testosterone levels can lose weight (Question 51); it's mostly due to loss of muscle mass. Check your thyroid function while you're at it with a TSH (thyroid-stimulating hormone) level.

3. *Depression.* This is a common cause of weight loss, because depressed people often lose their appetites (Questions 82 and 83).

4. *Lipoatrophy.* This doesn't usually cause loss of total body weight, but it can make you look like you've lost weight (Question 46).

5. *Gastrointestinal disorders.* Problems in the esophagus could make it harder to swallow; nausea and vomiting could make you less likely to eat or to absorb your food; you could also have a problem with absorption of nutrients in the small intestine.

In the past, we often used anabolic steroids to help people gain muscle mass as they wasted away from AIDS. It wasn't a solution to the problem, but it helped control the symptoms. We don't see wasting from AIDS anymore—in fact, obesity is a much bigger problem—but there are still people who want to take anabolic steroids to build up their muscles. Needless to say (but I'll say it anyway), this is not a good idea from a health standpoint. These steroids have other side effects, including liver damage, erectile dysfunction, and personality changes. You also could induce hypogonadism, as your own body's testosterone production will be suppressed.

70. Why am I tired?

Fatigue is common among people with HIV . . . and people without HIV, too, for that matter. Feeling tired is among the most common complaints in any medical practice, whether it involves HIV or not. If you're experiencing an unusual amount of fatigue, consider the following possible causes:

- *Depression.* This may be the most common serious reason for fatigue. People with depression have no energy, but they also have a number of other symptoms, discussed in Question 82.

- *Sleep apnea and other sleep disorders.* Not getting enough sleep at night will obviously make you tired and sleepy during the day. Sleep apnea, which is when people temporarily stop breathing at night, is much more common than we realized, especially if you're overweight. A clue might be that your partner tells you that you snore heavily or that you have prolonged periods at night where you appear to stop breathing. During this time, your oxygen level falls, triggering your body to briefly wake up—so sleep is not really restorative or restful. People with sleep apnea might also describe frequently falling asleep during the day. This problem can be diagnosed with a sleep study, which is fortunately now usually done at home. Besides sleep apnea, there are other causes of poor sleep, including excess caffeine or alcohol before bed, or intense television or video gaming, or simply having your phone with its alerts going off on your nightstand. Limiting these negative sleep factors is part of what's called "sleep hygiene" and is highly recommended!

- *Anemia.* In addition to fatigue, people with anemia may be pale, dizzy, and short of breath. Causes include medications, especially zidovudine (AZT, *Retrovir, Combivir, Trizivir*), dietary deficiencies, HIV-related complications, and HIV itself. Anemia is easy to diagnose with a simple blood count (done every 6 months when you are on ART), but further tests are then necessary to determine the cause.

- *Hormone deficiencies.* These include low testosterone levels (hypogonadism), thyroid hormone deficiency (**hypothyroidism**), and adrenal insufficiency (Question 51).

Hypothyroidism
A deficiency in thyroid hormone.

- *Medications.* Zidovudine is known to cause fatigue even when it's not causing anemia. Efavirenz (*Sustiva, Atripla*) can do it, too, especially in the first few weeks if it's disturbing your sleep with lots of wild dreams (Question 52). Some people on efavirenz have such vivid dreams that they feel, upon awakening, that they have been awake all night!

- *Lactic acidosis.* This is an uncommon but serious side effect of stavudine (d4T, *Zerit*), zidovudine, and possibly didanosine (ddI, *Videx*). Lactic acidosis causes other symptoms as well, which are discussed in Question 45. You shouldn't be on these medications.

- *HIV.* is common in people with high viral loads and/or low CD4 counts or when there's significant wasting.

Because virtually all of the medical causes of fatigue are treatable, it's important to make the diagnosis. Fatigue is not something you should have to live with.

71. Can HIV affect my skin?

Skin problems can be caused by HIV itself, by complications of HIV, and by medications. It's hard to talk about skin problems in a book with no color pictures. If you're having skin problems, see your provider or a dermatologist. Here's an incomplete list of things that can go wrong with the skin:

- **Abscesses** ("boils") are common may be due to community-acquired **methicillin-resistant *Staphylococcus aureus*** (**MRSA**). They usually have to be opened up and drained. It's important to culture the pus first so that the right antibiotic can be chosen.
- Drug reactions often begin with a red, itchy rash. They can be caused by the NNRTIs, some PIs, especially fosamprenavir (*Lexiva*) and darunavir (*Prezista, Prezcobix, Symtuza*), trimethoprim-sulfamethoxazole, and many other medications.
- **Folliculitis** causes raised, itchy, red bumps in areas where there's hair. It can be caused by bacteria, *Demodex* mites, or can be "eosinophilic," a term used to describe the type of cells that are seen on a biopsy.
- Herpes simplex can affect the lips, the genitals, the area around the anus, or other parts of the skin. It causes small, painful blisters that open up and become shallow ulcers on a red base.
- Kaposi's sarcoma causes raised purple lesions on the skin or in the mouth (Question 61).
- **Molluscum contagiosum** lesions are raised, skin-colored, fleshy bumps with small indentations

---

Anemia is easy to diagnose with a simple blood count.

Abscesses

Collections of pus (infectious organisms and white blood cells) in the skin ("boil") or other parts of the body.

Methicillin-resistant *Staphylococcus aureus* (MRSA)

A drug-resistant bacterium that traditionally caused serious illness in seriously ill, hospitalized patients but that has recently become a common cause of skin disease, including abscesses (community-acquired MRSA).

Folliculitis

Infection of the hair follicles and skin around them.

Molluscum contagiosum

Flesh-colored bumps or protuberances on the skin that are caused by a poxvirus and can be sexually transmitted.

in the middle. They can occur anywhere but are especially common on the genitals, face, and neck.

- Opportunistic infections can cause skin problems, including cryptococcosis, histoplasmosis, and *Bartonella* (**bacillary angiomatosis**). A skin biopsy is usually the best way to make the diagnosis.

- **Prurigo nodularis** sounds exotic, but it's just a way to say "itchy bumps" in Latin. This may be a reaction to too much scratching over a long period of time.

- **Psoriasis** can get worse or appear for the first time in people with low CD4 counts. It causes itchy raised patches, especially on the elbows, knees, and buttocks.

- **Scabies** is caused by a common skin mite. It causes intense itching, especially at night. A common location is on the backs of the hands and between the fingers. It can be severe in people with low CD4 counts.

- **Seborrheic dermatitis** causes a flaky, red rash on the face, especially in the folds on the cheeks and around the eyebrows.

- Secondary syphilis can cause a variety of rashes, including red bumps, sometimes involving the palms and soles (Question 89).

- Shingles is reactivation of varicella-zoster virus (VZV), the chickenpox virus, in the skin over a single nerve. It causes painful blisters in a confined, band-like area on one side of the body.

72. Why do I have a headache?

If your CD4 count is over 100 and you've got a headache, it's probably due to one of the usual causes—tension

Bartonella

A bacterium that can cause skin disease (bacillary angiomatosis) or liver disease (peliosis hepatis) in people with HIV.

Bacillary angiomatosis

A bacterial skin disease caused by *Bartonella*, which causes raised purple lesions on the skin; sometimes confused with Kaposi's sarcoma.

Prurigo nodularis

A condition characterized by itchy bumps on the skin, seen more commonly in people with HIV.

Psoriasis

A skin condition that results in dry, scaly, itchy plaques on the skin that can get worse with immunosuppression due to HIV.

Scabies

An itchy skin condition caused by a mite that burrows under the skin and can be spread to others by close contact.

Seborrheic dermatitis

A common skin condition causing flakiness on the face, especially around the eyebrows and in the folds on the cheeks.

Tension headache

A headache caused by muscle tension.

Migraine headache

A severe headache, often on one side of the head, sometimes accompanied by visual changes or nausea.

Sinus headache

A headache caused by congestion of the sinuses (see **Sinusitis**).

Listeria

A foodborne bacterium that can cause meningitis and other infections. Although not common, the risk for acquiring *Listeria* is higher in people with HIV.

headache, migraine, or sinus headache. A **tension headache** feels like a band-like tightness or constriction, tends to come on later in the day, and is present on both sides of the head. A **migraine headache** can occur at any time of the day, is often present on one side of the head, may be throbbing, and may occur with visual changes or nausea. People with a **sinus headache** have sinus congestion, a feeling of fullness or pressure below the eyes or in the forehead, and sometimes plentiful thick snot.

Some of our medications can cause headache, in particular zidovudine (*Retrovir, Combivir, Trizivir*) and the integrase inhbitors. Everyone knows that excess drinking can lead to heachaches the next day, and there isn't a coffee drinker in the world who has not experienced a caffeine withdrawal headache the first morning they miss their usual cup of coffee.

If your CD4 count is below 100 and you have a headache, especially a chronic headache that gets gradually worse, possibly with fever or stiff neck, you should be checked for cryptococcal meningitis (Question 57). A simple blood test, the serum cryptococcal antigen, will determine whether cryptococcal meningitis is likely. If the test is positive, you need an immediate spinal tap to confirm the diagnosis and to find out the severity. Other types of meningitis (bacterial, *Listeria*) are far less common but come on more suddenly. They can also start out with a headache and fever.

If you also have neurologic changes (seizures, weakness, or numbness on one side of the body; coordination problems; or mental changes), you could have a mass in the brain, usually caused by either toxoplasmosis (Question 56) or a brain lymphoma. The first step here is an MRI scan of the brain with contrast injected through the vein. Progressive multifocal leukoencephalopathy (PML), which is caused by **JC virus**, can also cause neurologic symptoms, but it's less likely to cause a headache.

73. Can HIV affect my nervous system?

Untreated HIV can wreak havoc your nervous system. The virus gets into the brain and spinal fluid and can lead to a lot of unpleasant complications, some of which are permanent. The way to prevent these problems is to take ART as soon after diagnosis as possible. I'll discuss the approach to some neurologic symptoms here:

- *Headache.* See Question 72.
- *Memory loss or personality changes.* The most common cause of memory loss is depression, which can sometimes look very much like dementia. It's possible to tell the difference with special memory and cognitive tests (**neuropsychological testing**), but if there's any question, a few weeks of treatment with an antidepressant may help sort it out (Questions 82 and 83). If you're experiencing memory loss but aren't depressed, then it's important to find out whether you have HIV dementia or other HIV-related brain complications.
- *Foot or leg pain or numbness.* The most common cause of peripheral neuropathy is toxicity from stavudine (d4T, *Zerit*) or didanosine (ddI, *Videx*). Untreated HIV can cause this too. The treatment is to start taking an ART regimen that doesn't include stavudine or didanosine (Question 45). Unfortunately, regardless of the cause, some cases of neuropathy are irreversible, even after stopping the offending medication or treating HIV.

If your CD4 count is below 100 and you have a headache, especially a chronic headache that gets gradually worse, possibly with fever or stiff neck, you should be checked for cryptococcal meningitis.

JC virus

The cause of progressive multifocal leukoencephalopathy (PML).

Neuropsychological testing

A series of tests, usually performed by a psychologist or neurologist, to assess memory and thinking skills. Can be used to diagnose dementia, or to determine whether someone has depression or dementia.

> The most common cause of memory loss is depression, which can sometimes look very much like dementia.

- *Seizures.* Anyone who has a seizure for the first time should go to an emergency room. A CT or MRI scan of the brain will be ordered to look for masses or lesions.

- *Weakness, coordination problems, unsteady gait, or incontinence.* Depending on the location of the symptoms, you will need an MRI scan of the brain and/or spinal cord

PART ELEVEN

Women's Issues, Pregnancy, and Children

How is HIV different for women?

What if I want to get pregnant?

What if my child is HIV positive?

More . . .

74. How is HIV different for women?

HIV in women is similar to HIV in men, but there are a few important differences. Women with HIV tend to have lower viral loads than HIV-positive men at the same CD4 counts. This shouldn't affect the decision of when to start treatment now that treatment is recommended for everyone.

Some studies suggested that women with HIV don't benefit as much from treatment as men, but that was because of delayed diagnosis, usually related to socio-economic factors and the fact that clinicians sometimes don't consider women at risk for HIV. In the United States, women at risk for HIV may have less access to health care; they are more likely to come from communities of color and to have lower annual incomes than men with HIV. If they were infected heterosexually, they may not realize they're at risk and avoid testing. But we know now that women who get diagnosed and treated for HIV live as long as men—longer, in fact, since women generally tend to outlive men.

Women respond well to ART. There are no HIV drugs that can't be used in women or that are specifically recommended for women, but there are some gender-specific issues to be aware of. Nevirapine (*Viramune*) is more likely to cause liver toxicity in women than in men, and it's not recommended for women starting treatment with CD4 counts above 250. While we don't recommend using nevirapine in anyone starting therapy these days, if you are taking it without problems you can continue, regardless of your sex or your CD4 cell count. We used to think that efavirenz (*Sustiva*, *Atripla*) could cause birth defects if given during the first trimester of pregnancy, but careful studies have not found this risk

(Question 76). There is now evidence that dolutegravir may be linked to a *small* increased risk in neural tube defects in babies if women conceive while receiving this drug. As a result, some providers might ask you to take other drugs when trying to become pregnant (such as raltegravir, or *Isentress*), but would not want you to choose something that is more toxic for you if dolutegravir is the best choice. A number of PIs and NNRTIs may decrease the effectiveness of birth control pills, making them unreliable. Women taking drugs that interact with birth control pills should use an additional form of contraception, such as condoms or a diaphragm.

Women respond well to ART. There are no HIV drugs that can't be used in women or that are specifically recommended for women.

75. Does HIV cause gynecologic problems?

A number of common gynecologic problems can be more frequent or severe in HIV-positive women. *Candida vaginitis* (a vaginal infection cause by *Candida*, a common yeast) is a good example. More recurrent or serious candidiasis is sometimes the first sign of immunosuppression in HIV-positive women. Vaginitis can be treated with topical antifungal agents or with oral fluconazole.

Bacterial vaginosis, a bacterial infection that causes vaginal discharge, is also more common in women with HIV. **Pelvic inflammatory disease (PID)**, an infection of the uterus and fallopian tubes usually caused by sexually transmitted infections, can sometimes be more serious and may be more likely to require surgery in HIV-positive women.

As in men, genital herpes can be more severe or recur more frequently as the CD4 count falls. It causes painful

Bacterial vaginosis

A bacterial infection of the vagina that causes vaginal discharge.

Pelvic inflammatory disease (PID)

A serious infection of the uterus and fallopian tubes usually caused by sexually transmitted infections, especially gonorrhea and chlamydia.

genital ulcers that should be treated with anti-herpes medications. Genital herpes can increase the viral load and can make it easier to transmit HIV. Women who have frequent herpes outbreaks should take daily medication to prevent flares. HIV-positive women can also develop idiopathic genital ulcers—ulcers for which no cause is found. These are similar to aphthous ulcers in the mouth and esophagus (Questions 64 and 65). They usually occur in women with very low CD4 counts and are best treated with ART, along with the advice of a gynecologist who is also an expert in treating HIV-positive women.

Human papillomavirus (HPV) (Question 81) causes genital warts, cervical dysplasia, and cervical cancer.

76. What if I want to get pregnant?

It is now standard of care that all women who are pregnant or planning to get pregnant should take an HIV test as soon as possible. The reason is that the earlier HIV is diagnosed and treated, the more effective medicine will be at preventing mother-to-child HIV transmission.

If you find out you have HIV, know that pregnancy is a completely realistic option now that we can treat HIV effectively and prevent infection in the baby. However, pregnancy should be carefully planned and monitored in women with HIV.

All pregnant women should be on ART, ideally starting before they become pregnant. ART is a *must* after the first trimester since transmission to the baby is extremely unlikely—essentially zero risk!—if Mom's viral load is undetectable at delivery. There are many recommended treatment options for pregnant women. The regimen should include a nucleoside pair, usually either *Truvada* or *Epzicom*. (Zidovudine/lamivudine is also on the recommended list, but pregnant women suffer from enough nausea already without having to suffer more on AZT!) This should be combined with either a boosted PI—either atazanavir (*Reyataz*) or darunavir (*Prezista*) boosted with ritonavir (*Norvir*)—or raltegravir (*Isentress*), the recommended integrase inhibitor. Once women are past the first trimester, they can also be on dolutegravir—it's only when dolutegravir was taken at the time of conception that a small risk to the baby was found.

We used to recommend elective cesarean section to further reduce the risk of transmission to the baby. However, we now know that if you are taking ART and have a suppressed viral load, this is no longer necessary.

If your partner is HIV negative, you should be on ART with an undetectable load before trying to conceive naturally, to protect him from infection. Short of that, you can use artificial insemination, either performed by a physician or at home using the "turkey baster" approach, in which the partner's semen is squirted into the vagina using a syringe to avoid intercourse. HIV-negative male partners could consider taking PrEP (Questions 13 and 86) while trying to conceive, though many experts (including me) think this is overkill if your viral load is undetectable.

HIV-positive women who want to get pregnant should talk to their provider and to an obstetrician-gynecologist with HIV expertise. There are many other issues to discuss besides ART, including safe conception, planning the delivery, breastfeeding, and medical care for the baby, just to name a few.

Pregnancy is a realistic option for women with HIV now that we can treat HIV effectively and prevent women passing it to the baby.

77. How can I father a child with an HIV-negative woman?

Having an undetectable viral load on ART is the most important thing you can do to prevent transmission. Studies show that it eliminates the risk entirely, though there are still some theoretical concerns—sometimes the virus is detectable in semen even when it's undetectable in the blood. Because of this concern, some women decide to take pre-exposure prophylaxis (PrEP) when they're trying to conceive with a partner who has HIV (Question 13).

Before we had the ability to fully suppress the viral load—and before we knew how effective it was at preventing transmission—some couples used **sperm washing**, which involves separating sperm from semen and inseminating the HIV-negative woman only with the sperm. The procedure is effective, but available only at a few medical centers and is very expensive. It is no longer necessary, and I don't recommend it for anyone.

Sperm washing

A technique in which sperm are separated from semen to lower the risk of HIV transmission to a woman during conception.

If your partner is taking ART with an undetectable viral load, and you're taking PrEP, you're already using the equivalent of a "belt and suspenders" to keep yourself from getting HIV. (I guess that's kind of a funny analogy in this context!) But if you're not comfortable relying entirely on these prevention benefits of an undetectable viral load, you can reduce the risk even further by timing intercourse with the most fertile part of your cycle using home ovulation tests.

If *both* partners are infected, conception can proceed the natural way provided both are on ART. Some of my patients have expressed concern about acquiring a "second strain" of HIV from sex with another positive partner.

However, this is not going to occur if both of you are on ART. And remember, the HIV status of the father is irrelevant as far as the baby goes because an infant can only be infected by its mother.

78. What if my child is HIV positive?

This book is written for HIV-positive adults, so a comprehensive review of childhood HIV is beyond the scope of what I can cover. Very simply, children and adolescents can get HIV either through **mother-to-child transmission** during pregnancy, labor, or breastfeeding. Fortunately this is completely preventable using ART during pregnancy and has become quite rare in the United States. Much more common today is an older child or adolescent getting HIV through sex or drug use. The same preventive strategies used for adults can be difficult to sustain in teenagers, as some do not engage consistently with health care.

Diagnosing babies is complicated because they carry the mother's HIV antibodies for up to 18 months, regardless of whether they're truly infected. It's passed along in the blood during pregnancy. Because the standard blood tests aren't helpful, **polymerase chain reaction (PCR)** testing of the blood is used to find the virus itself. Also, the CD4 counts that indicate immunosuppression in children under 5 are higher than those in older children and adults.

Without treatment, many HIV-positive babies get sick within the first year of life. More often, they do well initially for several years, not becoming ill until they enter pre-school or grade school. Untreated children with HIV may not gain weight or grow normally, and they

Mother-to-child transmission

Transmission of HIV from mother to infant during late pregnancy, labor, or breastfeeding.

Polymerase chain reaction (PCR)

A laboratory technique used to detect or quantify the DNA or RNA of an infectious organism for diagnostic purposes.

Diagnos-ing babies is compli-cated because they carry the mother's HIV anti-bodies for up to 18 months, regardless of whether they're truly infected.

may have neurologic problems that can cause delayed mental development, poor school performance, or cerebral palsy.

Treatment of children is similar to treatment of adults. However, not all drugs come in forms that kids can swallow, and there aren't as many studies on the treatment of children as there are for adults.

HIV-positive adolescents can be especially challenging . . . even more challenging than adolescents *without* HIV! Issues such as adherence, stigma, discrimination, disclosure, depression, drug and alcohol use, and the prevention of further transmission can be especially daunting at this stage of life. Adolescents with HIV need to be treated by providers who are experts both in HIV and adolescent medicine.

PART TWELVE

Coinfection

What if I also have hepatitis C?

What if I also have hepatitis B?

How do I prevent cervical and anal cancer?

More . . .

79. What if I also have hepatitis C?

Coinfection

The combination of two infections, such as HIV plus either hepatitis B virus or hepatitis C virus.

Cirrhosis

A form of permanent liver damage with many possible causes, most commonly alcoholism or chronic hepatitis.

Hepatocellular carcinoma (or hepatoma, or liver cancer)

Cancer of the liver that can be caused by alcoholism or chronic hepatitis.

Interferon

An injectable medication used in the past to treat hepatitis C and sometimes hepatitis B.

Direct-acting antiviral (DAA)

A hepatitis C treatment that works directly against the virus, to distinguish it from interferon, which needs your immune system to work. DAAs in combination can cure hepatitis C.

Coinfection with both HIV and hepatitis C virus (HCV) is common, especially among people who inject drugs, because both viruses are easily passed from one person to another with shared needles or syringes. Since people with HCV have more virus in their blood than people with HIV, HCV is more easily spread by sharing noodles than HIV. HCV can also be transmitted sexually, though not as easily as HIV and the hepatitis B virus (HBV), and mostly between men who have sex with men. HCV is a common cause of severe liver disease, including **cirrhosis** (liver scarring) and **hepatocellular carcinoma** (or **hepatoma**, or **liver cancer**). Now that people aren't dying of AIDS as often, HCV has become an increasingly important cause of death among people with HIV.

Untreated HIV can make hepatitis C get worse more rapidly. If you're coinfected with HIV and HCV, it's possible that ART will slow the progression of hepatitis. You should get vaccinated against the hepatitis A and B viruses if you're not already immune because those viruses can cause more severe disease in people with HCV infection.

Importantly, don't drink alcohol. Alcohol use, even in moderation, is a big risk factor for HCV progression.

Unlike HIV and hepatitis B, hepatitis C can be now be *easily cured.* The dreaded **interferon**, which caused fatigue and depression and a whole host of other nasty side effects, is no longer necessary. This has been replaced by pills called **direct-acting antivirals**, or DAAs. These DAAs are simple pills, taken once daily, and after a mere 2 to 3 months of therapy, they cure hepatitis C in nearly 100% of people!

Your provider can prove that you are cured of hepatitis C by checking your viral load 12 weeks after you stop treatment. If the viral load is undetectable, you can consider yourself cured. Importantly, just because you've been cured of hepatitis C doesn't mean you can't get it again. If you continue or resume the activities that gave you HCV in the first place, you can get hepatitis C again.

Treating hepatitis C is now much easier than treating common medical conditions such as arthritis, diabetes, and high blood pressure. The only difficult thing about treating and curing hepatitis C is getting the drugs paid for. The good news is that competition has brought down the prices substantially. It is now much easier to get HCV treatment covered by insurance than it was in 2014-2015, when these DAA treatments first became available.

If your HCV is managed by someone other than your HIV provider, make sure they communicate with each other. Some of the HCV drugs interact with antiretroviral medications. You may have to switch to a different ART regimen during treatment for HCV, in particular if your regimen contains the "boosters" ritonavir or cobicistat.

Hepatitis C comes in several related but genetically different types, called **genotypes**. (Think of them like different dog breeds.) Your provider can check your hepatitis C genotype with a simple blood test. With early HCV treatment, the genotype mattered a lot,

Genotype

The genetic composition of a virus. Used to describe related but genetically different types of hepatitis C. Can be checked with a simple blood test.

Now that people aren't dying of AIDS as often, HCV has become an increasingly important cause of death among HIV-positive people.

since the treatments worked better against some genotypes than others. But the latest advances with hepatitis C treatment are treatments that are **pan-genotypic**, meaning they treat all genotypes equally well.

The two pan-genotypic treatments for hepatitis C are sofosbuvir/velpatasvir (*Epclusa*) and glecaprevir/pibrentasvir (*Mavyret*). *Epclusa* is 1 pill daily for 12 weeks for everyone. *Mavyret* is 3 pills daily for 8 weeks for most patients. They have different drug interactions and slightly different side effects. But both treatments are nearly 100% effective for all genotypes, are very well tolerated, and easy to take. And best of all—once you're finished, your hepatitis C is cured!

80. What if I also have hepatitis B?

It's not unusual to be infected with both HIV and the hepatitis B virus (HBV), since both are spread in the same way (sex and blood exposure). Most people who are diagnosed with HBV clear the infection on their own, sometimes after getting sick with hepatitis, but sometimes without ever knowing they were infected. However, others never clear the infection and go on to develop chronic HBV infection, which can lead to chronic hepatitis, cirrhosis, or liver cancer. People with HIV are more likely to develop chronic hepatitis B than HIV-negative people.

Everyone with HIV should be tested for HBV, and vice versa. A negative hepatitis B surface antigen (**HBsAg**) generally means you don't have chronic hepatitis B. A positive hepatitis B surface antibody (**HBsAb**) means you've been exposed and are immune, either since you cleared it on your own or had a successful hepatitis B vaccine.

If your HBsAb and HBsAg are negative, you should be vaccinated with a series of three shots using the older hepatitis B vaccine, or two shots with the new vaccine. If your surface antibody and antigen are negative but your core antibody (HBcAb or anti-HBc IgG) is positive, you should still be checked for chronic hepatitis with an HBV DNA test, which is a hepatitis B viral load. If that's negative, you should be vaccinated. As with all vaccines, you're more likely to respond to the vaccine if you wait until after you've responded to HIV therapy.

People who have both HIV and HBV should always be treated for both infections at the same time because some HIV drugs are also active against HBV. Trying to treat just one without causing resistance in the other is difficult and involves taking less desirable medications. The easiest way to treat HIV/HBV coinfection is with an ART combination that contains either tenofovir DF or AF and either emtricitabine or lamivudine. Many of our combination therapies already include tenofovir and emtricitabine, so there are several excellent choices. Treatments that should be avoided in HIV and HBV coinfection only include lamivudine and emtricitabine *without* tenofovir, because these drugs on their own have a high risk of selecting for hepatitis B resistance.

People who have both HIV and HBV should be treated for both infections at the same time.

What if you can't take tenofovir? Then your provider should add another hepatitis B treatment to your HIV regimen, a medication called entecavir (*Baraclude*)

Stopping HBV drugs can lead to a dangerous flare of hepatitis. People with chronic HBV infection should also get checked periodically for cirrhosis and liver cancer with an ultrasound of the liver and the **alpha-fetoprotein (AFP)** blood test.

Alpha-fetoprotein (AFP)

A blood test used to look for liver cancer.

81. How do I prevent cervical and anal cancer?

Both cervical and anal cancer are caused by human papillomavirus (HPV), a sexually transmitted virus that first causes changes in the cells of the cervix and anus (**dysplasia**) that can later turn into cancer. HPV infection is common and so is dysplasia. Fortunately, anal and cervical *cancers* are much less common and can be prevented.

The cervical Pap smear is a routine test for women to look for cervical dysplasia. HIV-positive women should get a Pap smear regularly—at least once a year. An abnormal Pap smear is evaluated by **colposcopy**, where abnormal areas can be looked at more closely and biopsied. High-grade lesions can then be treated with minor surgery.

Because **anal dysplasia** is also caused by HPV, involves similar cells, and can also progress to cancer, many experts diagnose and treat anal dysplasia like they do cervical dysplasia, though the evidence supporting this approach is not as strong as it is for cervical cancer. That's now possible using an anal Pap smear and **high-resolution anoscopy** (HRA), the anal equivalent of colposcopy.

An anal Pap smear is a simple procedure: a wet swab is inserted in the anus and twisted around on its way out. But it doesn't make sense to do anal Pap smears unless there's someone trained to follow up the abnormal results with HRA, to biopsy suspicion lesions, and to treat high-grade lesions. Screening for anal dysplasia is mostly done in men who have had sex with men and in women; especially women who have cervical dysplasia

Dysplasia

Abnormal development or growth of tissues, organs, or cells.

Colposcopy

A procedure used to more closely examine the cervix for dysplasia due to HPV infection in women who have had abnormal Pap smears.

Anal dysplasia

Abnormal cells in the anus caused by HPV. If left untreated, it can progress to anal cancer.

High-resolution anoscopy (HRA)

A procedure used to more closely examine the lining of the anus for dysplasia due to HPV infection in people who have had abnormal Pap smears.

or anal or genital warts. Straight men can have anal dysplasia, too (even straight men who've never had sex with a man), so some argue that we should be doing this test in everybody.

There are now effective vaccines to prevent HPV infection, especially the strains that cause cancer (Question 26). It's approved for men and women up to the age of 26, but is best used in children or adolescents before they become sexually active. Young HIV-positive people should be vaccinated, and guidelines now note that if you are up to age 45 and want the HPV vaccine, you should get it!

PART THIRTEEN

Mental Health and Substance Use

How do I know if I'm depressed?

What should I do if I'm depressed?

What are the risks of using drugs if I have HIV?

More . . .

82. How do I know if I'm depressed?

HIV-positive people who are depressed may assume they're just having a normal response to having HIV. But depression, in the true medical sense of the word, is *never* "normal." People often describe themselves as being "depressed" when what they *really* mean is that they're sad, disappointed, angry, worried, or demoralized—perfectly normal responses to the bad things that happen to all of us in life.

Depression, on the other hand, is not a *normal* response to life's misfortunes. Some people can be depressed for no obvious reason when everything's going well objectively, while others experience terrible suffering without ever being depressed. While depression can be triggered by life events in people who are prone to it, the fact that you're depressed has to do with both brain chemistry and external circumstances. How much each one plays a role in a person's depression is different in each case.

People who are depressed feel sad, empty, hollow, hopeless, and isolated. Activities and people they once enjoyed no longer bring pleasure. They may lose interest in sex, work, hobbies, friends, and family. They see no light at the end of the tunnel—the future looks bleak. They may have insomnia, or they may sleep too much. They may lose their appetite for food or overeat. They may abuse drugs or alcohol or engage in high-risk sex because these activities provide momentary relief. Symptoms can include fatigue, weight loss (or gain), memory loss, and headache.

People who are depressed feel sad, empty, hollow, hopeless, and isolated. Activities and people they once enjoyed no longer bring pleasure.

In contrast, people who are experiencing normal coping problems—dealing with an HIV diagnosis, for example—may feel sad, stressed, angry, or worried, but they understand that they'll get through it. They can be "cheered up" or distracted by keeping busy, or by being with friends, or engaging in activities they enjoy.

If my description of depression rings true to you, talk to your medical provider immediately. Depression is a dangerous but highly treatable condition. It's also one of the biggest risk factors for poor adherence with antiretroviral medications—another reason to take it seriously.

83. What should I do if I'm depressed?

If you view depression as a normal emotion, a sign of weakness, or a character flaw, you won't get the help you need. Think of depression as though it were pneumonia. You *might* get better on your own, but it won't be pleasant. It could take a long time. It *could* even kill you. With treatment, things can get better quickly.

The best way to treat depression is to talk to a health care provider, who may recommend further counselling or that you take **antidepressants**—drugs that restore the normal balance of chemicals in your brain, which have become out of balance while you're depressed. There are many antidepressants available. They all work to treat depression but have different side effects. Some antidepressants are sedating, which can be helpful for people with insomnia. Others can perk you up if you're fatigued or sleeping too much. Some antidepressants can cause sexual side effects, especially delayed orgasm. Most antidepressants also help control anxiety and obsessive thoughts. One patient of mine, whose son had suffered greatly from complications of heroin addiction, told me that taking antidepressants for his depression made him ruminate less over his son's problems. He still

Antidepressants
Drugs used to treat depression.

Depression is a dangerous but highly treatable condition.

knew they were problems—they just didn't lead him to feel depressed and overwhelmed himself. The antidepressant treatment enabled him to get back to being productive at work and a good father to his son and other children.

When you take an antidepressant, don't expect sudden or dramatic changes. It can take 2 to 4 weeks before you start to notice a difference. The point isn't to change your personality or to make you ecstatically happy. The point of antidepressants is to make you feel like yourself again. Antidepressants won't change the circumstances of your life, but they can help you cope with those circumstances. They're not habit forming—they can be tapered and stopped when you no longer need them. (And it's important to taper most of them—suddenly stopping antidepressants can make you feel terrible. Your provider can give you guidance how to do this.) If you don't tolerate the first drug you try, don't give up. Switch to a drug with a different side effect profile.

The best way to treat depression is to take antidepressants—drugs that restore the balance of chemicals in your brain, which have become out of balance when you're depressed.

Counseling and psychotherapy can make medications more effective, and, in some people, make taking medications unnecessary. Talk therapy becomes especially useful as you start to get better—it helps you return to life, to deal with issues that might have contributed to your depression, and to keep you healthy after you get better. Psychotherapy is also great for people who aren't depressed but are having problems coping with life circumstances.

84. What are the risks of using drugs if I have HIV?

Before getting into what most people think of when they use the word "drugs," let me discuss the most commonly used drug of abuse in the United States—and that's alcohol. It's widely accepted that occasional or light alcohol use is generally safe (unless you have liver problems, including hepatitis C—then no alcohol is safe). However, excess alcohol use has numerous negative medical and psychological consequences, many of them no doubt already known to you (Question 92).

How do you know if your drinking is a problem? One simple way is to see if it's negatively influencing your relationships with partners, friends, or family; if it's reducing your performance at work or in family responsibilities; or if you notice health issues that you attribute to your drinking. If you are answering "yes," or even "maybe" to any of these questions, you have a problem with alcohol and should get help. Your provider will be able to refer you to available services in your area to help with alcohol addiction.

Now, onto the other drugs. People with HIV often assume that drug use is bad for them because it lowers their CD4 count and increases their viral load. But that's not the reason to stay away from drugs. Still, there are plenty of great reasons to stay away from drugs.

First, there are the medical dangers of the drugs themselves. Cocaine causes heart attacks and mental illness. Injecting heroin or other drugs can lead to serious bacterial infections of the heart valves, bones, and joints—in fact, these infections are now a greater risk to people who inject drugs than HIV and hepatitis C. I have seen many young people permanently disabled, or even die, from these infections. Methamphetamine can destroy your teeth, your brain, your relationships, your career, and your life.

All of the drugs I just mentioned are addictive. Early on, people might have a tendency to believe they can keep use of cocaine, heroin, and crystal meth under control. But once you start using, you are at great risk of needing to increase the dose and frequency until they start interfering with your life—your relationships with partners, friends, and family, and your work life. Everything starts to take a back seat to the addiction.

It's hard to come up with too many dire warnings about the dangers of marijuana, which is now legal in many states. But even its advocates admit that regular heavy use can make you dumb and lazy, and there's now some evidence that it could increase the risk of mental illness later in life. There is evidence that *Aspergillus*, a fungus that can cause dangerous infections in people with very low CD4 counts, can live in marijuana leaves and can be inhaled. (If you smoke dope and have a low CD4 count, we used to recommend microwaving the joint to kill the fungus. Please don't ask which setting to use or for how long—those studies will never be done!)

Aspergillus

A fungus that causes aspergillosis, a potentially serious infection involving the lungs that can occur in people with very advanced HIV disease.

Drugs can also interact with your HIV medications. Drug companies don't typically study interactions between their drugs and illegal substances, but there is evidence that people have been harmed by taking "club drugs," such as MDMA (*Ecstasy*) and ketamine, along with antiretrovirals, for example.

Drug use can increase your risk of getting other infections or of spreading HIV to others. If you've got a drug problem, get treatment before you start ART.

Drug use can increase your risk of getting other infections or of spreading HIV to others. Being high lowers your inhibitions and clouds your judgment, allowing you to take risks that you wouldn't otherwise take, putting you at risk for sexually transmitted diseases, including syphilis (Question 89) and hepatitis C (Question 79). Injection is especially risky, since it can spread HIV, hepatitis C, and other bloodborne infections.

Finally, studies show that active drug users are less likely to take ART correctly, putting them at risk of HIV drug resistance and losing treatment options. If you've got a drug problem and starting ART isn't urgent, get treatment before you start. Don't wait until you've messed up and developed drug resistance.

Ultimately, the best reason to stay away from drugs is to keep yourself physically and mentally healthy so you'll have the upper hand against HIV.

PART FOURTEEN

Relationships, Sexuality, and Prevention

How and when should I disclose my HIV status to partners?

How do I have safe sex?

What should I know about sexually transmitted infections?

More . . .

85. How and when should I disclose my HIV status to partners?

Having HIV doesn't mean you can't have intimate relationships or sex. But even in the era of "U = U," where people on ART with undetectable viral loads won't transmit the virus to their partners, I still think you should disclose your HIV status.

Some argue that disclosure isn't necessary if you're practicing safe sex or are on ART. They point out that everyone knows the risks and should be protecting themselves, regardless of what their partners say—or don't say—about their status. There are also situations where disclosure is unrealistic. Anonymous sex taking place in a bathhouse or dark alley rarely involves a "How do you do?" much less a detailed exchange of medical information. Then again, someone having sex in that environment should assume a high level of risk and take the appropriate precautions.

Disclosure becomes especially important when you're dating or starting a new relationship. Some deal with this by dating only HIV-positive partners. That simplifies things, but it's not possible for everyone. Disclosing your status to a negative partner can sometimes be a deal breaker, resulting not only in rejection but also—in the worst-case scenario—the risk that your new "ex" may share your information with others. For that reason, many choose to wait until there's mutual affection, trust, and a sense that the relationship is going somewhere.

The problem is that the longer you wait, the more likely your new partner will feel betrayed when you finally disclose your status, especially if the relationship has already become sexual. In addition, put yourself in their place—wouldn't you want to know your partner's status, if for no other reason but for it to be an expression of honesty and trust in the relationship? If you're positive and your goal is to be in a relationship, you may have to take things a bit slower than when you didn't have HIV. Get to know and trust your partner first, talk about your HIV status later, and *then* have sex. If this process takes a while, remember that in Jane Austen novels, couples didn't even use first names until the engagement was announced, and holding gloved hands was evidence that things had progressed to an advanced level of intimacy!

86. How do I have safe sex?

There is no sexual activity that is guaranteed not to transmit HIV, and there's at least *some* risk involved in most activities—at least the most popular ones. I can't give you odds or percentages, since the risk depends not only on what you're doing, but on how you're doing it and your viral load. The risk is essentially eliminated if the viral load is undetectable. In studies looking at "discordant couples" (couples in which one is positive and the other is negative), we have seen *no* cases of transmission when the positive partner has an undetectable viral load—even when the couples are specifically recruited because they're not using condoms. Important message—being on effective ART is *the* most effective way to prevent transmission during sex.

But let's imagine that your viral load is higher than 200 and you're not on ART. (Note—you should be.) Here are some general comments about the "riskiness" of the more common sexual activities, assuming the viral load is detectable and condoms aren't being used:

- *Anal and vaginal intercourse.* If the positive partner is on top, this is the highest-risk activity.

A condom reduces the risk dramatically if it doesn't break. The risk is much lower if the positive partner is on the bottom. That's because the lining of the anus and vagina is made of **mucosal cells**, which can be infected, whereas the penis is almost completely covered by skin, which can't. However, a man can still get infected from being on top. The risk is higher if he's uncircumcised or has herpes, syphilis, or other open sores on his penis. The risk of spreading both HIV and the hepatitis C virus increases if there's bleeding during sex.

- *Oral sex.* HIV can be transmitted by getting a positive person's preseminal fluid ("pre-cum"), semen ("cum"), vaginal fluid, or menstrual blood in the mouth. (It has nothing to do with swallowing because the stomach is an inhospitable place for viruses to survive.) The risk is higher if the gums are in bad shape. If the positive partner is giving oral sex to the negative partner, there's essentially no risk of HIV transmission, though other STIs can be spread that way.

- *Oral-anal sex ("rimming").* You won't spread HIV this way, but the person doing the rimming could get hepatitis A or a bacterial or parasitic gastrointestinal infection.

- *Mutual masturbation.* This is very safe as long as you don't have open cuts or sores on the hands and keep fluids out of the mouth and eyes.

- *"Water sports."* Urine is a safe bodily fluid.

- *Kissing, hugging, cuddling, massage.* All safe.

87. What if my partner is negative?

Let's assume that disclosure is out of the way (Question 85). You're positive, and your negative partner knows it. What next?

Mucosal cells

Cells that line the internal organs and body orifices, such as the mouth, nostrils, anus, and genital area.

It's your responsibility to make sure you never infect *anyone,* including your negative partner. "This infection stops with me" are words to live by. Of course, HIV-negative adults should be aware of the risks and should be protecting themselves as well. Unfortunately, that approach hasn't been working, and the U.S. epidemic continues at a rate of about 40,000 new cases per year. Prevention experts are now changing the prevention message to focus on those who are positive—people who know better than anyone how important it is to prevent transmission and who must bear most of the responsibility for not spreading the infection.

People who don't have HIV sometimes make crazy choices and stupid decisions. Some may seem perfectly willing to put themselves at risk of infection. It's the moral obligation of the positive partner not to cooperate with that kind of self-destructive behavior, to ensure that their HIV is never transmitted. We live in a community and should watch out for each other.

The most important thing you can do to prevent transmission to a negative partner is to maintain an undetectable viral load on ART, the most effective form of prevention we have. As I've already said (numerous times, but it's important!), that's all you need, especially if you've been "undetectable" for years and get your labs checked regularly.

But for some HIV-negative people, that may not be enough, which is their choice. They may still want to use condoms, especially for high-risk activities or to prevent other sexually transmitted infections. In some cases, they may choose to use PrEP for greater piece of mind. Even though they don't need it to prevent getting HIV from you, I wouldn't refuse to prescribe PrEP to someone who strongly wanted it. That person may just want it for extra security—or they may be having sex outside the relationship and not want to disclose this. (Yes, this happens.) For more on the relative risk of various sexual activities, see Question 86.

88. What if my partner and I are both positive?

Superinfection

Reinfection with a new strain of HIV in someone who has already been infected.

Recombinant strains

Strains of HIV that are combinations of two or more other strains.

Subtypes

In the case of HIV, groups of related viruses, also called "clades" or "sub-clades." Most HIV-positive people in the United States are infected with subtype B, but there are many other subtypes throughout the world.

Superinfection can cause a rise in viral load and a drop in CD4 count, similar to what happens with initial infection.

Being with a positive partner eliminates concerns about new HIV transmission, but there are still reasons to consider protected sex, including avoidance of other sexually transmitted infections (Question 89). Back before we recommended that all people with HIV be on ART, we also used to worry about something called **superinfection**. If you and your partner are not on ART, it's possible to be superinfected with additional strains of virus. There have been some well-documented cases, which also explains why there are **recombinant strains** of HIV in the world (viruses that are combinations of two or more **subtypes**). As noted, superinfection has not been reported in people on ART, and I suspect it will never happen! In other words, two people with undetectable viral loads don't have to worry about superinfection.

When talking to my patients about sex with other positive partners, I recommend condoms with casual partners, mainly to prevent sexually transmitted infections. In steady relationships, the decision to abandon condoms will depend primarily on whether each partner is on ART with an undetectable viral load and whether they're monogamous. If one has hepatitis C, condoms should be used until that is treated and cured.

89. What should I know about sexually transmitted infections?

Becoming positive doesn't mean you can stop worrying about sexually transmitted infections (STIs). There are others to be avoided.

Syphilis can be worse in people with HIV. It can progress more rapidly if it's not treated. It's more likely to infect the nervous system and can affect your vision and hearing. The blood tests we use to monitor your response to syphilis treatment can be harder to interpret and can take longer to become negative than in HIV-negative people. If you're HIV positive, you should be checked for syphilis, and the test should be repeated at least once a year—more often if you're sexually active with multiple partners.

Gonorrhea and **chlamydia** are common infections that can infect the urethra of the penis, the cervix, the anus, and the throat. Gonorrhea has become resistant to standard oral antibiotics and must now be treated with an injection. (In fact, if things keep going the way they're going with drug resistance, we may eventually need to treat gonorrhea with intravenous therapy.) Men with HIV should be checked for gonorrhea and chlamydia with a urine test and also with anal and/or throat swabs if they're having anal and/or oral sex; women should be tested at the time of their routine pelvic exam. A different type of chlamydial infection, **lymphogranuloma venereum** (**LGV**) sometimes causes anal and rectal infections (**proctitis**) in gay men. It tends to be more severe than standard chlamydia and takes longer to treat. I hear gay men tell me they've been "tested for STDs," but all they've had is a syphilis blood test and a urine test, which only looks for gonorrhea and chlamydia in the urethra of the

Syphilis
A sexually transmitted infection caused by *Treponema pallidum*, a bacterium, that can cause anal, genital, or mouth lesions (primary syphilis); fever, rash, and hepatitis (secondary syphilis); or infection of the brain, spinal fluid, eyes, or ears (neurosyphilis). It can also be dormant, causing no symptoms (latent syphilis).

Becoming positive doesn't mean you can stop worrying about sexually transmitted infections.

Gonorrhea
A sexually transmitted infection caused by the bacterium *Neisseria gonorrhoeae*.

Chlamydia
A sexually transmitted infection caused by *Chlamydia trachomatis*.

Lymphogranuloma venereum (LGV)

A sexually transmitted infection caused by *Chlamydia*.

Proctitis

Infection or inflammation of the rectum.

penis. If you're having oral and anal sex and no one has swabbed your throat and butt, you've haven't been thoroughly tested.

Genital herpes, usually caused by herpes simplex virus type 2 (HSV-2), causes painful blisters and shallow ulcers on the genitals, around the anus, or on the skin. The infection persists for life and can recur, especially in people with low CD4 counts. ART can help, but outbreaks should be treated with an anti-herpes medication, such as acyclovir, famciclovir, or valacyclovir. If you're having frequent outbreaks, you should take one of those medications daily, which not only prevents herpes flares, but also the risk of herpes (and possibly HIV) transmission.

Human papillomavirus (HPV) infection is discussed in Questions 26 and 81. There are other STIs that I haven't discussed but that are also best avoided.

PART FIFTEEN

Living with HIV

What foods and water are safe?

Should I take vitamins or supplements?

Can I travel abroad?

More . . .

90. What foods and water are safe?

There are few foods you should *avoid* eating because of HIV, but there are some guidelines to follow, especially if your CD4 count is low. This advice applies particularly if you have just been diagnosed, and your immune system has not yet had a chance to improve on ART.

Avoid undercooked meat (beef, lamb, pork), especially if your *Toxoplasma* antibody is negative (Question 56). Avoid raw eggs, undercooked poultry, unpasteurized milk or fruit juices, and raw sprouts—hey, this is good advice for *everyone*, not just for people with HIV. Hard cheeses (like cheddar) are safer than soft cheeses (like brie, feta, Camembert, or Mexican cheeses), which may contain *Listeria*, a bacterium that can cause meningitis (though not often). Avoiding raw shellfish is a good idea, but if you can't resist a raw oyster, make sure you're immune to hepatitis A (Question 26). Some doctors recommend avoiding sushi, but that seems cruel and extreme to me since the parasites you can get from sushi aren't worse if you have HIV than if you don't. Be careful not to "cross-contaminate" food when you're preparing it. For good food safety tips, check out www.foodsafety.gov.

What *should* you eat? Healthy food, preferably *real* food: food that you or someone else cooks from original, pronounceable ingredients. *Eat Real Food, Not Too Much, Mostly Plants*, is the title of a book I strongly recommend written by Michael Pollan. It's a fun book to read about how to eat in a healthy way, but if you don't have the time, the title says it all! Eat fresh fruits and vegetables—with every meal, every day. Starches should be brown, not white—the white, refined starches just get turned into sugar. Think of dessert as a special treat, not a daily course. Avoid too many packaged foods, those bright-colored indestructible products that have lists of ingredients a mile long. Given the choice be-tween an apple—a real apple—and an apple-flavored, pre-packaged item in a shiny package, go with the for-mer every time, even if the latter claims to have all sorts of "healthy" additives.

To gain weight, eat more—preferably high-calorie nat-ural foods such as nuts, sauces with olive oil, and small portions of meat, fish, or chicken. To lose weight, eat less. Break the rules once in a while, but not every day. When you *do* break the rules, break them without guilt. Finally, before you develop too many rigid dietary rules or restrictions, remember that eating is not a form of medical therapy but one of life's great pleasures.

What about water? For most HIV-positive people, tap water is perfectly safe. If you're young and not familiar with the term "tap water," it refers to a plentiful, healthy beverage that people used to drink *directly from faucets and drinking fountains without charge*, but that has been replaced by an expensive, bottled version that I call "tap water from a city you don't live in." How millions of gullible Americans were duped into voluntarily hand-ing over money to large corporations for something that is still free is a great mystery, but it happened—the discarded plastic evidence of it is everywhere.

The best reasons to pay for water are if your tap water tastes bad, is known to be of bad quality, or if you like it fizzy. (And note that excessive, long-term consump-tion of fizzy beverages, including water, may decrease bone density.) Otherwise, tap water is fine for most people. If your CD4 count is below 100, be aware of the risk of **cryptosporidiosis**. *Cryptosporidium* is a parasite that can be passed from person to person or ingested in contaminated water. Tap water is usually safe, but there

Cryptosporidiosis
Diarrhea caused by *Cryptosporidium*, a parasite that can be found in contami-nated water or trans-mitted from person to person.

have been occasional outbreaks when the water supply becomes contaminated. You can protect yourself by filtering tap water through a 100-micron filter. Bottled water is OK, too, but only if the company filters it in the same way, which is not guaranteed.

91. Should I take vitamins or supplements?

Unless you suffer from a known nutritional deficiency, or have problems with your intestines that keep you from absorbing real food, vitamins and supplements are worthless. Actually, they're worse than that—several studies evaluating the health effects of vitamins have sometimes surprisingly found health *harms* from vitamins. Not only that, they are often expensive, and some can even interfere with proper absorption of food and medicines.

Diagnoses of "vitamin D deficiency" have been all the rage over the past decade or more, and as a result many people are taking vitamin D supplements, sometimes along with calcium. While it's true many of us have low vitamin D levels—especially in the winter, since we get lots of our vitamin D from sunlight—there is very little evidence that vitamin D supplements actually help anyone. Much better would be to increase your intake of leafy green vegetables and other vitamin D rich foods. Also, if the weather is fine, go outside and get some exercise in the sunshine! Even those calcium supplements some people have been taking for years to keep bones strong have been shown to have negative effects, in particular triggering kidney stones. They might even be bad for your heart. One other problem with calcium is that it interferes with your body's ability to absorb integrase inhibitors. So if you must take calcium, be sure to separate it from your ART regimen by at least a couple of hours.

92. Can I still drink alcohol?

The answer depends on whether it would have been OK for you to drink if you were HIV negative. HIV itself has very little to do with it. First, let's talk about who should *not* drink:

1. People with chronic hepatitis B or C shouldn't drink because it can make the hepatitis worse and increase the risk of cirrhosis (see Questions 79 and 80). After you've been cured of hepatitis C, you can consider drinking in moderation, provided you don't have cirrhosis.

2. People with alcoholism shouldn't drink because few are capable of drinking in moderation. Excessive alcohol consumption is bad for just about every organ in your body. It is especially bad for your liver, which may already be stressed by some of the medications we use to treat HIV. There are other conditions that can be caused by both alcohol abuse and by either HIV or ART, including neuropathy, dementia, blood disorders, heart problems, and pancreatitis, just to name a few. Why increase your risk? Finally, people who are drunk are lousy medication takers, and we've already talked about what happens when you don't take your medications (Question 31). If you're wondering whether you have a problem with alcohol, there's a good chance you do. If alcohol has repeatedly caused problems with your work, relationships, or criminal or driving record; if you can't control your drinking; if

Crypto-sporidium *is a parasite that can be passed from person to person or ingested in contaminated water.*

other people think you drink too much; if you feel guilty or lie about your drinking; or if you wake up hungover or shaky until you get an eye-opener, then you've got a problem, one that needs to be addressed sooner rather than later.

If you can drink in moderation and have no medical reason to avoid alcohol, then drinking is OK with HIV and with HIV medications.

If you can drink in moderation and have no medical reason to avoid alcohol, then drinking is OK with HIV and with all HIV medications. Alcohol does not interfere with the activity of the medications or increase their toxicity, as long as you're not overdoing it. Keep it down to a maximum of two drinks per day: two glasses of wine, two beers, or two ounces of hard liquor. And if you don't drink all week, that doesn't mean you can have 14 drinks on Friday night!

93. Can I travel abroad?

Yes, but there are a few things to consider, especially if you're going to a resource-limited country where there are infections you wouldn't normally come in contact with. If your CD4 count is over 200, the risk is about the same as it would be for anyone else. But if your count is low, especially less than 50, then you should avoid travel of all sort and focus on the single most important thing about improving your health—getting on effective ART so that your immune system improves. You can travel once this occurs, and it won't take long!

The CDC website (www.cdc.gov/travel) has excellent country-specific information about precautions and vaccinations. People with HIV who have low CD4 counts (less than 200) should generally avoid vaccines that contain live viruses or bacteria. This is especially true for oral **typhoid vaccine** (get the injectable vaccine instead). If **yellow fever** vaccine is required and your CD4 count is low, consider going to Orlando rather than Ouagadougou. Getting the vaccine is fine if you have a high CD4 count and there's a definite risk of yellow fever where you're going. Make sure you've had a tetanus booster in the last 10 years and have been vaccinated against hepatitis A and B if you're not already immune (Question 25). Take the usual precautions to avoid travelers' diarrhea, and talk to your doctor about bringing an antibiotic along to treat it if it happens.

No matter where you're going, make sure you have enough meds for the entire trip and then some. Plan ahead for cancelled or delayed flights—they happen! Bring the original bottles to avoid problems at the airport, and carry them on the plane rather than checking them in your luggage. If you're going on a very prolonged trip, check with your pharmacy about getting a bigger supply of medications than usual. Often insurance plans will allow this for travel.

I generally don't recommend travel to people who were just diagnosed and who have advanced HIV with low CD4 cell counts. They should stay close to home and concentrate on getting healthy and starting ART. However, sometimes travel is unavoidable. If this is your situation, I recommend asking your provider for the name of an HIV doctor or clinic in the area you are traveling to, just in case a complication happens. You probably won't need it, but it never hurts to have this information!

94. Can I have pets?

Several studies have shown that having pets is associated with greater happiness and life satisfaction—one recent paper even found an association with prolonged

Typhoid vaccine

A vaccine to prevent typhoid fever, a bacterial infection of the blood caused by *Salmonella typhi*, sometimes acquired by travelers to developing countries.

Yellow fever

A serious disease caused by yellow fever virus, which is transmitted by mosquitoes and sometimes acquired by travelers to parts of Africa or Latin America.

HIV-positive people should generally avoid vaccines that contain live viruses or bacteria.

survival! The good news is that you can still have pets if you follow a few simple precautions. And remember that most of the concerns and precautions pertain to people with low CD4 counts and are not on ART— once you get on treatment, your immune system will be strong enough to have any domestic pet.

If possible, stay away from very young animals (less than 6 months old), and avoid contact with sick animals. Pets with diarrhea should get checked for bugs in their feces that could be passed on to you. Wash your hands well after handling your pets and before eating.

Cats can carry *Toxoplasma gondii,* the parasite that causes toxoplasmosis (Question 56), which you get from eating cat poop. *"But I don't eat cat poop!"* you protest. These things can happen, usually if you've been changing a litter box and get it on your hands and then in your mouth. Assuming you're not already infected (find out whether you have a positive *Toxoplasma* antibody), the best solution is to get someone else to change the litter box. If you and Kitty live alone together, then wear gloves, wash your hands, and change the box every day because it's harder to get toxo from fresh poop. Indoor kitties are safer than the outdoor prowlers. Take the same precautions with gardening, too.

Cats can also transmit *Bartonella,* the bacterium that causes cat-scratch disease in children as well as bacillary angiomatosis (a skin disease) and **peliosis hepatis** (an infection of the liver) in people with HIV who have very low CD4 cell counts (less than 100). Older cats are safer than young ones. Don't play rough with Kitty. (As a cat owner myself, this is good advice for everyone—my cat Otto can be quite fickle and has even swiped my wife, the person who loves him the most.)

Peliosis hepatis

An uncommon liver infection caused by *Bartonella.*

Fortunately, pet-related infections are uncommon, and are treatable conditions—not a justification for declawing your cat as a preventative measure. Sorry, but you can't use HIV as an excuse to save your sofa!

Reptiles, chicks, and ducklings can carry *Salmonella,* a bacterium that causes diarrhea and other problems, and people with HIV are particularly vulnerable. Wash well after handling Mr. Lizard or consider trading him in for a different animal. There have also been reports of *Salmonella* in common pet treats, so don't share them with your animals—not that you were thinking of doing that, right?

What about dogs? My dog Louie is an absolute sweetheart. (Can you tell I love him more than our cat Otto?) However, dog behavior is quite variable, so approach strange dogs with caution. Dog and cat bites should be attended to promptly, as they have a high risk of getting infected. Wash them thoroughly with soap and water, and if they are quite deep or painful, get evaluated by a clinician so that you can start antibiotics.

95. Can I still exercise?

You can and you should! Mainly because it's a healthy way to live, and it's important to maintain your overall health if you're HIV positive. But there are some reasons to exercise that are specific to HIV as well:

1. Some of the older antiretroviral drugs can cause fat accumulation, insulin resistance, and elevations in cholesterol and triglycerides (Questions 43 and 46), which in turn can increase the risk of heart disease, and some people who are now on newer agents are stuck with these problems

from drugs they took in the past. Aerobic exercise helps to reverse all of those conditions. Even our current safer treatments sometimes lead to weight gain. After starting treatment, some of this weight gain is a return to health—the virus has made you lose weight. But after a while, this weight gain can overshoot what is healthy. A combination of exercise and diet is the best way to avoid gaining too much weight.

2. Although we don't know the cause, we're seeing loss of bone density in people with HIV (Question 50). Exercise, especially resistance exercise, can help to maintain bone density.

3. Some of the older antiretroviral drugs caused lipoatrophy (fat loss) involving the legs, arms, and buttocks (Question 46). Resistance training can increase the muscle mass in these areas, which can help to compensate for the loss in fat.

4. Some HIV-positive people are at greater risk for depression. Exercise is a great natural antidepressant.

If you're not used to exercising, start slow. Walk more. Take the stairs. Park in the far corner of the lot. Over half the car trips made in the United States daily are under a mile—consider walking instead! If you're a fair-weather walker, join a gym. Don't do the same type of exercise each day, but mix it up so you don't get bored. Exercise with a friend, or listen to music or a recorded book. If you're someone who likes the exercise bike or elliptical, and are having trouble sticking with it, use this time to catch up on a Netflix series or watch music videos on YouTube. A slug-like existence may be more likely to kill you than HIV, so *don't be a slug!*

96. What are advance directives?

To overstate the obvious, *Everybody dies.* Whether you have HIV, some other chronic disease, or are the picture of health, you will someday take your last breath. Before we had effective treatment for HIV, an untimely death from AIDS was a virtual certainty. We HIV doctors used to spend a lot of time discussing with our patients how they wanted to spend their final days, weeks, and months, hoping for the best possible death. It was a very sad, but necessary, conversation.

Today, we spend more time talking about life, old age, and retirement. But getting older is a great reminder that we still need to make plans for when we are one day unable to care for ourself or are facing serious medical problems that could be fatal. The best time to think about these things is when you're healthy and have no immediate plans to leave the planet.

What kind of medical care would you want if you were sick and unable to make decisions for yourself? Would you want life-sustaining measures—to be resuscitated with **CPR** or to be put on a breathing machine in the intensive care unit—if the chances of recovery were low? Would you want any treatment at all, including artificial feeding, if you had a terminal illness? Who would you choose to make medical decisions for you?

If you know the answers to these questions, you need **advance directives**—legal documents that make your wishes known to others in case you can't speak for yourself. A **living will** is a legal document that lets you spell out the medical treatments and life-sustaining measures you would want or not want if you were unable to make those decisions for yourself. A living will is

CPR

Cardiopulmonary resuscitation. Procedures used to try to revive someone whose heart has stopped and/ or has stopped breathing.

Advance directives

Legal documents that allow you to make decisions about end-of-life care ahead of time (see **Living will** and **Durable power of attorney for health care**).

Living will

A legal document that allows you to state which medical procedures and life-sustaining measures you would want if you were no longer able to make decisions for yourself.

important, but it's not enough because it doesn't cover every decision that might need to be made. It's even more important to choose the person who would make medical decisions for you if you couldn't make them for yourself. If that person is your legally recognized spouse, then you're covered, because your spouse is automatically your next of kin. But if you want decisions to be made by an unmarried partner, a friend, or a different family member, then you need to appoint that person using a **durable power of attorney for health care**, a legal document that trumps next-of-kin rules, and your living will, too, for that matter. This document also allows your partner or friend to visit you in the hospital if visitation is otherwise limited to immediate family members. The person you appoint should be aware of your wishes in advance—including what's in your living will—and should agree to act in accordance with those wishes.

Durable power of attorney for health care

A legal document that allows you to authorize someone else to make medical decisions on your behalf if you lose the ability to make decisions for yourself.

Everyone should have these documents. You don't need a lawyer—the forms are available online and in most clinics and hospitals. Give a copy to your provider and to the person you've named as your decision maker.

You should also have a will, especially if you want your belongings to go to someone other than your immediate family members. Whether you'll need a lawyer to draw up a will depends on how complex your finances and your wishes are. Simple wills can be drafted using software programs.

No one likes to think or talk about dying, but the consequences of not having advance directives can be tragic. Make your wishes known, and make them count!

PART SIXTEEN

Questions for Those Who Still Have Questions

What about the theory that HIV doesn't cause AIDS?

Isn't it true that drug companies are withholding the cure to make money?

What's the state of the global epidemic?

More . . .

97. What about the theory that HIV doesn't cause AIDS?

In the early years of the AIDS epidemic, shortly after the discovery of HIV, a few scientists questioned whether AIDS was really caused by HIV. They proposed a number of alternative explanations, suggesting that AIDS was caused by illegal drug use and zidovudine (in the developed world) and malnutrition (in the developing world). These scientists argued that **Koch's postulates** had not been fulfilled and warned that antiretroviral therapy, rather than saving lives, was prematurely ending them.

Koch's postulates

The four criteria needed to prove that a microbe or organism is the cause of a disease. The postulates are: (1) the organism must be found in all animals suffering from the disease but should not be found in healthy animals; (2) the organism must be isolated from a diseased animal and grown in pure culture; (3) the cultured organism should cause disease when introduced into a healthy animal; and (4) the organism must be reisolated from the experimentally infected animal.

If their hypothesis was far-fetched in the late-1980s, it's complete lunacy today. Koch's postulates have been fulfilled many times over. We now have a solid and ever-growing understanding of how HIV infects human cells, damages the immune system, and causes AIDS. The life-saving effects of ART have been well established by countless clinical trials, large observational studies, and data from large populations. It was no accident that the death rate from AIDS declined by 50% in the year after effective therapy was introduced. And if HIV didn't cause AIDS, how could we now expect life expectancy on ART to be as long for a healthy person with HIV as a similarly aged person who is HIV negative?

The few so-called "scientists" who cling to their discredited hypotheses have forgotten one of the fundamental principles of science: You have to be able to admit that you might be *wrong*. Their dwindling followers (most have either died prematurely or have come to their senses and started therapy before it was too late) now treat "HIV denialism" more as a religious cult than as a scientific hypothesis. These people would be amusing if it weren't for their influence—in many ways the equivalent of the anti-vaccine activists whose beliefs are truly harmful to individual and public health alike.

HIV denialists influenced the policies of the South African government for many years. The tragic irony is that this country has had the worst HIV epidemic in the world for many years. These policies resulted in years of preventable deaths and new infections, and they have influenced gullible people to refuse an effective treatment for a fatal disease. Fortunately, ART is now widely available in South Africa, where they have more people on HIV treatment than any other country.

98. Isn't it true that drug companies are withholding the cure to make money?

This is a popular point of view among conspiracy theorists, in particular those with contempt for drug companies. A little rational thought should put this myth to rest:

1. It's no surprise that we haven't yet cured HIV. The difficulty of finding a cure is discussed in Question 42.

2. People who develop therapies at drug companies are scientists. They're motivated by the things that motivate scientists everywhere else: publication in prestigious journals, the respect of their colleagues, Nobel Prizes, TV interviews, getting funding to do more research, and the knowledge that their work has made a difference to humankind. No scientist who discovers the cure for AIDS is going to keep quiet about it.

3. Drug companies are competitive. If they're onto something big, their competitors can't be far behind. No company strives to be the *second* company with The Cure. If a company had a cure, you'd have heard about it. Take a look at the hepatitis C example—scientists and drug companies competed for years to find an interferon-free cure for hepatitis C, ultimately succeeding in 2014.

4. A cure for AIDS will be highly profitable. Sure, there's profit in lifetime therapy, too, but it's shared among multiple competing drug companies and doesn't last forever. Drugs go off patent and get replaced by generics; they fall out of favor as they're replaced by newer and better agents. Again, the hepatitis C example is pertinent—the companies that had successful DAAs that replaced interferon made an enormous amount of money. A cure for HIV would be highly profitable too!

5. *Most* conspiracy theories are wrong.

99. How do we know HIV wasn't created in a lab?

This popular conspiracy theory gives *way* too much credit to the science of bygone generations. HIV first infected humans in the first half of the 20th century. We have proof of human infection dating back to the 1950s, and it probably became a human disease several decades before that. The idea that such a complex virus could be created by scientists today is far-fetched enough, but to think that it could have been invented 80 years ago is preposterous.

Few of those who believe in this theory think it was just an innocent scientific experiment gone wrong. Instead, they think it was part of a well-orchestrated plot to rid the country—or the world—of its "undesirable elements": gay men, injection drug users, or minorities . . . take your pick. But in the 1930s we were worried about poverty; in the 1940s, it was the Germans and Japanese; and in the 1950s and 1960s, it was the communists. No one had the time or resources to think about wiping out gay men and drug users, who were barely on the radar screens of anyone except *other* gay men and drug users.

The fact that the HIV epidemic didn't originate in the developed world—where, as we know, all the Evil Scientists live—doesn't fit well with this theory either.

Because the epidemic began in Africa, you'd have to propose that someone was trying to wipe out all Africans, a strategy that would not have been appreciated by the colonial powers who relied on them for labor and income.

Finally, it's inconceivable that the inventor of such a virus could have planned an epidemic that would target specific groups of people. Its spread among gay men, drug users, and minorities was accidental, and of course it didn't stay confined to those groups. Throughout history, there have been infamous examples of abuse of the human race by science and medicine, but the deliberate creation of the HIV epidemic is *not* one of them.

100. What's the state of the global epidemic?

If you're reading this book, you probably live in a place where treatment is available and affordable. The global epidemic is more challenging. More than 35 million

Throughout history, there have been infamous examples of abuse of the human race by science and medicine, but the deliberate creation of the HIV epidemic is not one of them.

people have died of AIDS, and more than 36 million are now living with HIV, most of them in resource-limited countries, especially in sub-Saharan Africa. In the early 2000s, it wiped out hard-earned economic and health-care gains in many developing countries, drastically reducing life expectancy and creating millions of orphans, whose prognosis is grim regardless of their HIV status.

The news hasn't been *all* bad. In about 2000, the developed world finally recognized that it couldn't go on ignoring the devastation in the poorer parts of the world, and money began flowing from the government, private, and philanthropic sectors to provide life-saving treatment for people throughout the world, or at least in those countries where there was a political will to deal with the AIDS epidemic. Generic drugs made treatment more affordable.

The global financial crisis threatened the progress that had been made, and although the economy has now improved in the United States, the commitment of our country and the other wealthy countries of the world depends very much on the whims of politicians. Viral load and resistance testing are often too expensive, and fewer drugs are available, so options are limited if the first regimen fails. Nonetheless, HIV treatment in the developing world has saved countless lives, and new infections are declining almost everywhere.

The fact that we have turned the corner on the HIV epidemic in many regions that previously had no treatment means we can end this book on a hopeful note. We know how to prevent, diagnose, and treat HIV, even without an available HIV vaccine or a cure. If enough people with HIV have access to ART, and stay on it indefinitely, new diagnoses will continue to fall—and this global epidemic will end. As someone who witnessed the terrible days when HIV caused countless and heart-breaking premature deaths, I can emphatically state that that day can't come soon enough.

But until then—and until we have a cure—continue taking care of yourself because you have a long life ahead of you!

Additional Resources

Consider this book just a starting point for learning about HIV. There are numerous excellent resources available on-line, and I've listed many of my favorites below. Note that there is also a tremendous amount of misinformation too, and I've done you the favor of *not* listing these sites. If you want to hear more from me – on a whole range of topics – I've been writing a blog for *NEJM Journal Watch* since 2009 called "HIV and ID Observations" (blogs.jwatch.org/hiv-id-observations). It includes further discussions of many of the HIV-related topics we've reviewed here, plus a bunch of other stuff (general infectious disease topics, miscellaneous medical issues, and pictures of my dog Louie). If that's not enough, here are some more sites to keep you busy:

Websites
- *AIDS.gov.* Basic information on HIV and on U.S. government strategy and programs: http://aids.gov/.
- *AIDSinfo.* A site of the U.S. Department of Health and Human Services (HHS), where you can find the latest guidelines, drug information, and news about clinical trials: www.aidsinfo.nih.gov.
- *AIDS InfoNet.* A project of the New Mexico AIDS Education and Training Center that provides information on HIV treatment and prevention in multiple languages: www.aidsinfonet.org.
- *AIDSmeds.* A good source of information about HIV treatment: www.aidsmeds.com.
- *American Academy of HIV Medicine.* You can find information about HIV providers in your area: www.aahivm.org. Note that the listing is not comprehensive.
- *AmfAR (American Foundation for AIDS Research).* Provides information on HIV, including research developments: www.amfar.org.
- *AVERT.* Domestic and international HIV information, news, and stories: www.avert.org.

- *BETA (Bulletin of Experimental Treatments for AIDS)*. A bulletin published by the San Francisco AIDS Foundation covering new developments in HIV therapy: www.sfaf.org/hiv-info/hot-topics/beta/.
- *The Body*. A patient-oriented site that provides updated information, coverage of new scientific findings, and answers to users' questions: www.thebody.com.
- *CDC National Center for HIV/AIDS, Viral Hepatitis, STD, and TB Prevention*. CDC website with basic HIV information and data on the U.S. epidemic: www.cdc.gov/nchhstp/.
- *ClinicalTrials.gov*. A source of up-to-date information about federally and privately supported clinical research studies, including trials of HIV therapies: www.clinicaltrials.gov.
- *GMHC (Gay Men's Health Crisis)*. A New York–based, patient-oriented website that provides basic HIV information and news: www.gmhc.org.
- *HIV InSite*. HIV information from the University of California, San Francisco: http://hivinsite.ucsf.edu/.
- *HIV Drug Interactions*. A site maintained by pharmacy experts at the University of Liverpool providing accurate information about what medications can be taken safely with ART. www.hiv-druginteractions.org
- *HIV Medicine Association*. Part of the Infectious Diseases Society of America, it has another HIV provider directory that compliments AAHIVM. www.hivma.org/hiv-provider-directory.
- *National AIDS Treatment Advocacy Project (NATAP)*. Continuously updated source of information on new scientific data on HIV and hepatitis C, including studies presented at scientific conferences: www.natap.org.
- *New York State Department of Health AIDS Institute*. Provides general information about HIV/AIDS: www.health.state.ny.us/diseases/aids/.
- *Positively Aware*. A magazine for HIV-positive people, that includes updates on drug development and scientific developments: http://positivelyaware.com/.
- *POZ*. An online and print magazine for people with HIV: www.poz.com.
- *Project Inform*. An organization that provides updated information about HIV treatment: www.projectinform.org.
- *TPAN*. A magazine for HIV-positive people, that includes updates on drug development and scientific developments: www.tpan.com.

Glossary

A

Abscesses: Collections of pus (infectious organisms and white blood cells) in the skin ("boil") or other parts of the body.

Acquired immunodeficiency syndrome: *See* **AIDS**.

Acute (or **primary**) **HIV**: The stage of HIV that occurs shortly after infection. At this stage, the viral load is very high. People often have symptoms during this stage.

Acute retroviral syndrome (ARS): A collection of symptoms, such as fever, rash, and swollen lymph nodes, that most people experience during primary infection, shortly after they're infected.

Acyclovir: A drug used to treat herpes simplex and varicella-zoster virus.

ADAP: *See* **AIDS Drug Assistance Program**.

Adherence (or **compliance**): The term used to refer to a patient's behavior with respect to following treatment recommendations, including taking medications, keeping medical appointments, etc.

Adrenal glands: Glands in the abdomen that produce cortisol, a steroid hormone that is essential to many bodily functions, including the response to stress.

Adrenal insufficiency: A deficiency in the amount of cortisol produced by the adrenal gland.

Advance directives: Legal documents that allow you to make decisions about end-of-life care ahead of time (*see* **Living will** and **Durable power of attorney for health care**).

Advanced HIV disease: The most advanced stage of HIV, usually in people with CD4 counts below 50 or 100.

Aerosolized pentamidine: *See* **Pentamidine**.

AIDS: Acquired immunodeficiency syndrome, a more advanced stage of HIV, defined by having a CD4 count below 200 or one of a list of AIDS-indicator conditions.

AIDS case definition: The criteria used by the Centers for Disease Control and Prevention (CDC) to classify someone as having AIDS (*see* **AIDS**).

AIDS-defining condition: *See* **AIDS-indicator condition**.

AIDS Drug Assistance Program (ADAP): A federally funded program that provides antiretroviral medications and other HIV-related medications to those who have no other way to pay for them. The programs are administered by the states, and coverage varies from state to state.

AIDS-indicator condition (or AIDS-defining condition): One of a list of conditions, including opportunistic infections and malignancies, that is used by the CDC to determine who has AIDS.

AIDS-related complex (ARC): An old term, no longer in use, for the stage of HIV disease in which people have symptoms but have not yet developed AIDS. Now referred to as "symptomatic HIV."

AIDS service organization (ASO): An organization that provides services to people with HIV.

Alpha-fetoprotein (AFP): A blood test used to look for liver cancer.

Alternative medicine: The use of a non-standard medical treatment in place of standard therapy.

Amphotericin B: An intravenous drug used to treat serious fungal infections.

Anal cancer: Cancer of the anus caused by human papillomavirus (HPV).

Anal dysplasia: Abnormal cells in the anus caused by human papillomavirus (HPV). If left untreated, it can progress to anal cancer.

Anal Pap smear: A diagnostic test to screen for anal dysplasia. Also called "anal cytology."

Anemia: A deficiency of red blood cells, usually diagnosed by a low hemoglobin or hematocrit on a complete blood count.

Angular cheilitis: Cracking of the corners of the lips, sometimes caused by *Candida*.

Anoscopy: *See* **High resolution anoscopy**.

Anti-CMV IgG antibody test: A blood test used to look for infection with CMV.

Anti-HBs: *See* **HBsAb**.

Antibodies: Proteins used by the immune system to fight infection. Antibodies are formed after exposure to antigens—foreign substances such as viruses or bacteria.

Antidepressants: Drugs used to treat depression.

Antigens: Proteins from organisms, such as bacteria or viruses, that stimulate an immune response.

Antiretroviral therapy (ART): Drug therapy that stops HIV from replicating and improves the function of the immune system.

Anti-*Toxoplasma* IgG antibody test: A blood test used to look for exposure to the *Toxoplasma* parasite.

Aphthous ulcers: Painful ulcers in the mouth (aphthous stomatitis) or esophagus (aphthous esophagitis) that can occur in people with HIV. The cause is unknown.

ARC: *See* **AIDS-related complex**.

ART: *See* **Antiretroviral therapy**.

Aseptic meningitis: Meningitis that is not caused by a bacterium that can be grown in culture. Can be caused by viruses (including HIV during acute retroviral syndrome) or drugs.

Aspergillus: A fungus that causes aspergillosis, a potentially serious infection involving the lungs that can occur in people with very advanced HIV disease.

Asymptomatic HIV: An early stage of HIV in which infected people have a positive test but no symptoms.

Atovaquone: A drug used to treat or prevent PCP, sold under the trade name *Mepron*.

Attachment: The first stage of entry, in which the virus binds to the CD4 receptor. Attachment inhibitors would block this step, though none is currently approved.

Avascular necrosis: Painful joint damage caused by osteonecrosis, usually affecting the hips but sometimes the shoulders.

Azithromycin: An antibiotic that can be used to treat or prevent MAC as well as some bacterial lung infections.

B

Bacillary angiomatosis: A bacterial disease of the skin caused by *Bartonella*, which causes raised purple lesions on the skin; sometimes confused with Kaposi's sarcoma.

Bacterial vaginosis: A bacterial infection of the vagina that causes vaginal discharge.

Bactrim: *See* **Trimethoprim-sulfamethoxazole**.

Bartonella: A bacterium that can cause skin disease (bacillary angiomatosis) or liver disease (peliosis hepatis) in people with HIV.

Bell's palsy: A paralysis of one side of the face that can be caused by a variety of infections, including actute HIV.

Benzodiazepine: A class of drugs used to treat anxiety and insomnia. Diazepam (*Valium*) and alprazolam (*Xanax*) are well-known examples. The drugs can be habit-forming and can interact with some antiretroviral drugs.

Bilirubin: A pigment produced in the liver. When bilirubin levels get too high, the skin and eyes can turn yellow ("jaundice" or "icterus"). Elevated bilirubin can be caused by hepatitis or by two antiretroviral drugs: indinavir (*Crixivan*) or atazanavir (*Reyataz*).

Biopsy: A procedure in which a piece of tissue is removed, either with a needle through the skin, through a scope placed in the lungs or gastrointestinal tract, or by a surgical procedure. The specimen is then examined under the microscope and/or submitted for culture to make a diagnosis.

Blip: A single detectable viral load with undetectable viral loads before and after.

Boosted protease inhibitors: These combine a protease inhibitor (PI) with cobicistat or with a low dose of ritonavir (*Norvir*), another PI that is used only to increase drug levels and prolong the half-life of other PIs.

Bronchitis: An infection of the bronchi (airways), usually caused by a viral infection, often after a common cold.

Bronchoscopy: A diagnostic procedure in which a flexible tube is inserted into the lungs through the mouth (under sedation) so that samples or biopsies can be taken.

Bronchospasm (or **reactive airways**): The tendency of the bronchi (airways in the lung) to constrict (narrow), causing shortness of breath or cough. This can be chronic (in patients with asthma, for example) or temporary, following an upper respiratory infection.

Burkitt's lymphoma: A type of lymphoma that is seen more frequently in people with HIV but is less common than non-Hodgkin's lymphoma (NHL).

C

Candida: A fungus (yeast) that can cause thrush, esophagitis, and vaginitis in people with HIV.

Candidiasis: An infection caused by *Candida*, a common yeast.

Case manager: A person who helps coordinate your medical care, provides referrals for needed services, and determines whether you qualify for any assistance or entitlement programs.

CBC: *See* **Complete blood count**.

CCR5: *See* **Coreceptors**.

CCR5 antagonist: A drug that blocks CCR5.

CD4 cell: A type of lymphocyte (a type of white blood cell) that can be infected by HIV. CD4 cells fight certain infections and cancers. The number of CD4 cells (CD4 count) declines with untreated HIV, which leads to immunosuppression.

CD4 count (or **CD4 cell count**): A lab test that measures the number of CD4 cells in the blood (expressed as number of cells per cubic millimeter). The CD4 count is the most important measure of immunosuppression and is the most important indicator of the need for treatment.

CD4 lymphocyte (or **CD4 cell or T-helper cell**): *See* **CD4 cell**.

CD4 percent: The percentage of lymphocytes that are CD4 cells. The CD4 percent is provided whenever a CD4 count is ordered and provides additional information about the state of the immune system.

CD4 receptor: A protein on the surface of the CD4 cell that the virus attaches to before entering the cell.

CD8 cells (or **CD8 lymphocytes, or T-suppressor cells**): Another type of lymphocyte affected by HIV. Measuring CD8 cells is not necessary, as the CD8 count is not used to make treatment decisions.

CD8 lymphocytes: *See* **CD8 cells**.

CDC: *See* **Centers for Disease Control and Prevention**.

Cellular immune system: The part of the immune system most directly affected by HIV. It controls a variety of bacterial, viral, fungal, and parasitic infections.

Centers for Disease Control and Prevention (CDC): A branch of the federal government, within the U.S. Department of Health and Human Services (HHS), that is charged with tracking, preventing, and controlling health problems in the United States, including infectious diseases such as HIV.

Cervical cancer: Cancer of the cervix (the mouth of the uterus) caused by human papillomavirus (HPV).

Cervical dysplasia: Abnormal cells of the cervix, the mouth of the uterus, caused by human papillomavirus (HPV). If left untreated, it can progress to cervical cancer.

Chemokines: *See* **Coreceptors**.

Chickenpox: *See* **Varicella-zoster virus**.

Chlamydia: A sexually transmitted infection caused by *Chlamydia trachomatis*.

Cholesterol: A substance found in body tissues and the blood. Cholesterol is ingested (in meat or animal products) and also manufactured by the body. Cholesterol levels are measured by blood tests.

Cirrhosis: A form of permanent liver damage caused by alcoholism or chronic hepatitis.

Clarithromycin: An antibiotic that can be used to treat or prevent MAC as well as some bacterial lung infections.

Clinical trial: A study in which a treatment for a medical condition is tested in human volunteers to determine the safety and/or effectiveness of the treatment. In the case of HIV, this could include the study of investigational or approved drugs. In a randomized trial, two or more treatments are compared, and the treatment is selected by random chance. In a double-blind trial, neither the subject nor the investigator knows which treatment the subject is receiving. In a placebo-controlled trial, a drug is compared against an inactive substance that is identical in appearance. In a multicenter trial, the same trial is conducted simultaneously at multiple centers, sometimes in multiple countries. Phase I trials evaluate safety and drug levels and help to determine a dose range in a small number of volunteers who may be HIV positive or negative. Phase II trials are conducted in a larger number of subjects, looking at both safety and effectiveness, often of several doses of the medication. Phase III trials are large studies conducted at multiple sites that are designed to find out whether the treatment is effective and to collect more safety information. Phase IV trials occur after a treatment is already approved to find out more about its effectiveness, safety, and the best way to use it.

Clotrimazole troches: Antifungal lozenges used to treat thrush.

CMV: *See* **Cytomegalovirus**.

Coccidioidomycosis ("valley fever"): A disease caused by *Coccidioides* *immitis*, a fungus found mostly in the deserts and valleys of the south-western United States and north-ern Mexico. It can cause lung disease, meningitis, and infection of other organs.

Cocktail: An outdated term for an antiretroviral regimen (combination of antiretroviral drugs).

Coinfection: The combination of two infections, such as HIV plus either hepatitis B virus or hepatitis C virus.

Colitis: Infection or inflammation of the colon (large intestine).

Colonization: The presence in the body of microorganisms (viruses, bac-teria, etc.) that are not causing symp-toms or disease.

Colonoscopy: A medical procedure in which a flexible scope is inserted into the rectum and colon through the anus, while the patient is sedated, in order to look for abnormalities and take biopsies.

Colposcopy: A procedure used to more closely examine the cervix for dysplasia due to human papillomavi-rus (HPV) infection in women who have had abnormal Pap smears.

Combination antiretroviral therapy (cART): Another term for "HAART."

Combination therapy: The use of more than one antiretroviral drug to suppress HIV.

Complementary and alternative medicine (CAM): Medical products or treatments that are not standard of care (*see* **Alternative medicine** and **Complementary medicine**).

Complementary medicine: The use of a non-standard medical treatment in addition to standard therapy.

Complete blood count (CBC): A standard blood test that measures the red and white blood cell counts, hema-tocrit, hemoglobin, and platelet count.

Compliance: *See* **Adherence**.

Comprehensive chemistry panel: A standard blood test that measures kidney function, looks for evidence of liver disease, assesses nutritional sta-tus, and looks for electrolyte (sodium, potassium) abnormalities.

Coreceptors (or **chemokines**): Pro-teins on the surface of the CD4 cell and other cells that the virus binds to after attaching to the CD4 receptor but before entering the cell. There are two coreceptors: CCR5 and CXCR4.

Cortisol: The steroid hormone pro-duced by the adrenal gland essential to many bodily functions, including the response to stress.

Cotrimoxazole: *See* **Trimethoprim-sulfamethoxazole**.

CPR: Cardiopulmonary resuscitation. Procedures used to try to revive some-one whose heart has stopped and/or has stopped breathing.

Cross-resistance: Resistance to one drug that results in resistance to other drugs, usually in the same class.

Cryptococcal antigen: A lab test performed on either blood or spinal fluid used to diagnose cryptococcal meningitis.

Cryptococcal meningitis: Meningitis (infection of the spinal fluid and spinal cord lining) caused by *Cryptococcus*.

Cryptococcus: A fungus or yeast that is a common cause of meningitis in people with HIV.

Cryptosporidiosis: Diarrhea caused by *Cryptosporidium*, a parasite that can be found in contaminated water or transmitted from person to person.

Cryptosporidium: The parasite that causes cryptosporidiosis, which can cause chronic diarrhea in immunosuppressed people. The organism can be found in contaminated water or transmitted from person to person.

Cushing's syndrome: Excessive cortisol levels either because of overproduction by the adrenal glands or use of steroid medications.

CXCR4: *See* **Coreceptors**.

Cytomegalovirus (CMV): A virus that can infect the eyes, the gastrointestinal tract, the liver, and the nervous system in people with advanced HIV. The most common cause of retinitis (infection of the back of the eye).

D

Dapsone: A drug used to treat or prevent PCP and to prevent toxoplasmosis.

Delta 32 deletion: A genetic condition resulting in the absence of CCR5 coreceptor on the CD4 cell.

Individuals who are heterozygous for this deletion (the mutation is present in only one copy of the gene) can be infected by HIV but progress more slowly. Those who are homozygous (the mutation is present in both copies of the gene) cannot be infected by R5 virus, the most common form of circulating HIV.

Detectable: A word used to describe a viral load that is high enough to be measured by a viral load test. A detectable viral load is one that is above 20 to 75, depending on which test is being used.

Detoxification: The removal of toxic substances from the body. An important function of the liver and kidneys.

Diabetes: A disorder resulting in elevated amounts of glucose (sugar) in the blood and urine.

Differentiation Assay: A confirmatory antibody test that detects whether HIV antibody is present and whether the antibody is to HIV-1 or to HIV-2.

Direct-acting antiviral (DAA): A hepatitis C treatment that works directly against the virus, to distinguish it from interferon, which needs your immune system to work. DAAs in combination can cure hepatitis C.

Directly observed therapy (DOT): A program in which treatment is given to a patient directly by a healthcare professional, at home or in a clinic, in order to ensure that it's taken. Most common with treatment for tuberculosis but sometimes used for HIV therapy.

Disclosure: The process of revealing your HIV status to others.

Drug classes: Categories or groups of HIV drugs that are classified based on the way the drugs work and the stage of the viral life cycle that they target.

Drug holiday: An old term for an interruption in therapy, usually when the decision was made by the patient.

dT: *See* **Tetanus toxoid**.

Durable power of attorney for health care: A legal document that allows you to authorize someone else to make medical decisions on your behalf if you lose the ability to make decisions for yourself.

Dysphagia: Difficulty swallowing.

Dysplasia: Abnormal development or growth of tissues, organs, or cells.

E

EBV: *See* **Epstein-Barr virus**.

EIA: *See* **Enzyme-linked immunoassay**.

ELISA: *See* **Enzyme-linked immunoassay**.

Elite controllers: HIV-infected people whose CD4 counts remain high and whose viral loads are undetectable without treatment.

Encephalitis: An infection of the brain.

Endoscopy: A medical procedure in which a flexible tube is inserted into the esophagus and stomach through the mouth, while the patient is sedated, in order to take samples or biopsies or to treat a variety of conditions.

Enteritis: Infection or inflammation of the small intestines.

Entry: The process by which HIV enters human cells.

Entry inhibitors: Drugs that block entry of the virus into the CD4 cell.

Envelope: The outer surface of the HIV virus.

Enzyme-linked immunoassay (ELISA or EIA): Traditionally, the initial antibody test used to diagnosed HIV. Positive tests were confirmed with Western blot assays.

Enzymes: Proteins that carry out a biological function. Examples of enzymes carried by HIV include reverse transcriptase, integrase, and protease. Each plays a role in allowing the virus to reproduce, and each is a target for antiretroviral therapy.

Epidemic: The appearance of new cases of disease (especially an infectious disease) in a human population at a higher rate than would be expected.

Epstein-Barr virus (EBV): A herpesvirus that causes infectious mononucleosis ("mono"), oral hairy leukoplakia, and some lymphomas.

Erythematous candidiasis: An infection of the mouth caused by *Candida* in which the roof of the mouth (palate) becomes red and sometimes painful.

Esophagitis: Infection or inflammation of the esophagus.

Esophagus: The tube that connects the mouth and throat to the stomach.

Ethambutol: A drug used to treat MAC and TB in combination with other drugs.

F

Failure: Loss of activity of ART. Includes virologic failure (detectable viral load on therapy), immunologic failure (falling CD4 count on therapy), and clinical failure (worsening symptoms on therapy).

Famciclovir: A drug used to treat herpes simplex and varicella-zoster virus.

Family Medical Leave Act (FMLA): A federal law that allows people to take time off work without fear of termination or loss of benefits to deal with their own serious or chronic medical problems or those of their family members. People who need this protection must file paperwork with their employers in advance.

Fasting glucose: Measures blood glucose levels after hours without food.

Fat accumulation (or **lipohypertrophy**): A component of the "lipodystrophy syndrome" in which fat accumulates in abnormal parts of the body, such as inside the abdomen, around the neck, in the breasts, or on the upper back at the base of the neck ("buffalo hump").

Flu: *See* **Influenza**.

Fluconazole: A drug used to treat fungal infections.

Flucytosine (5FC): A drug used to treat fungal infections, usually in combination with amphotericin.

FMLA: *See* **Family Medical Leave Act**.

Folinic acid: *See* **Leucovorin**.

Folliculitis: Infection of the hair follicles and skin around them.

Fourth-generation HIV tests: HIV tests that detect both antigen and antibody, allowing them to detect HIV sooner after infection than older antibody tests.

Fusion: The final stage of viral entry in which the envelope of the virus fuses (merges) with the membrane of the cell, allowing entry of the virus into the cells. A fusion inhibitor blocks this process.

G

Gastritis: Infection or inflammation of the stomach.

Gastrointestinal: Relating to the GI tract: esophagus, stomach, small intestines, colon, and rectum.

Genotype: The genetic composition of a virus. Used to describe related but genetically different types of hepatitis C. Can be checked with a simple blood test.

Genotype tests: In HIV, a type of resistance test that looks for specific resistance mutations known to cause resistance to antiretroviral drugs.

Gonorrhea: A sexually transmitted infection caused by the bacterium *Neisseria gonorrhoeae*.

gp120: The part of the envelope (outer surface) of HIV that binds to receptors on the surface of the CD4 cell, allowing entry into the cell.

Guillain-Barré syndrome: Progressive muscle paralysis starting in the legs and moving upward, sometimes seen during acute retroviral syndrome.

H

HAART: *See* **Highly active antiretroviral therapy**.

Half-life: The amount of time it takes for the blood levels of a drug to decline by 50% after the last dose. Drugs with longer half-lives remain in the blood longer and can be taken less often.

HAV antibody: A blood test for hepatitis A. The IgM antibody tests for acute hepatitis A. The total or IgG antibody tests for prior infection or vaccination.

HBsAb (or **anti-HBs**): A blood test to determine immunity to hepatitis B. A positive result means you're immune to the hepatitis B virus either because of prior infection or vaccination.

HBsAg: A blood test to diagnose acute or chronic hepatitis B. A positive result means there is active hepatitis, but it doesn't distinguish between acute and chronic hepatitis.

HBV DNA: The "viral load" for hepatitis B, used to make the diagnosis in some people with negative HBV antibodies and to monitor response to hepatitis B therapy.

HCV RNA: The "viral load" for hepatitis C, used to confirm the diagnosis in people with a positive HCV antibody, to make the diagnosis in some people with a negative antibody, and to monitor response to hepatitis C therapy.

Hematocrit: A measure of the amount of red blood cells in the blood. (*See* **Complete blood count** and **Anemia**.)

Hemoglobin: The oxygen-carrying component of red blood cells. Also used as a measure of the amount of red blood cells in the blood. (*See* **Complete blood count** and **Anemia**.)

Hepatic steatosis ("fatty liver"): A buildup of fat in the liver that can be caused by a variety of medical conditions. When caused by antiretroviral agents, it is often accompanied by lactic acidosis.

Hepatitis: Inflammation or infection of the liver.

Hepatitis A: A viral infection of the liver caused by hepatitis A virus (HAV). It is spread by ingestion of feces or of food or water contaminated by feces. Unlike hepatitis B and C, hepatitis A never causes chronic infection.

Hepatitis B: A viral infection of the liver caused by hepatitis B virus (HBV). Like HIV, it is spread sexually, through exposure to infected blood or at childbirth. A proportion of people with HBV infection can develop chronic hepatitis and liver disease.

Hepatitis C: A viral infection of the liver caused by hepatitis C virus (HCV). It is spread primarily through exposure to blood (injection drug use or occupational exposures) but can also be transmitted sexually. Hepatitis C commonly causes chronic infection.

Hepatocellular carcinoma (or **hepatoma,** or **liver cancer**): Cancer of the liver that can be caused by alcoholism or chronic hepatitis.

Hepatoma: *See* **Hepatocellular carcinoma.**

Hepatotoxicity: *See* **Liver toxicity.**

Herpes simplex virus (HSV): A virus that causes painful blisters and ulcers on the lips, genitals, near the anus, or other parts of the skin.

Herpes zoster: *See* **Shingles.**

Herpesvirus: A family of viruses that can cause acute infection but that also remain latent in the body and recur. Examples of herpesviruses include herpes simplex virus (HSV-1 and HSV-2), varicella-zoster virus (VZV), cytomegalovirus (CMV), Epstein-Barr virus (EBV), and human herpesvirus-8 (HHV-8).

HHV-8: The virus that causes Kaposi's sarcoma, Castleman's syndrome, and some rare lymphomas. Also called Kaposi's sarcoma–associated herpesvirus (KSHV).

Highly active antiretroviral therapy (HAART): Antiretroviral therapy meant to suppress the viral load to undetectable levels, using a combination of several agents to prevent resistance (now usually just referred to as antiretroviral therapy [ART]).

High-resolution anoscopy (HRA): A procedure used to more closely examine the lining of the anus for dysplasia due to human papillomavirus (HPV) infection in people who have had abnormal anal Pap smears.

Histoplasmosis: A disease caused by *Histoplasma capsulatum*, a fungus found mostly in the Ohio and Mississippi River valleys, which causes lung infection in people with normal immune systems and infection of the lungs and other organs in people with low CD4 counts.

HIV: Human immunodeficiency virus, the virus that causes HIV and AIDS.

HIV-1: The most common form of HIV worldwide.

HIV disease: The name for the disease caused by HIV. AIDS is a late stage of HIV.

HIVAN: *See* **Nephropathy, HIV-associated.**

HLA B*5701: A blood test used to predict the likelihood of the abacavir hypersensitivity reaction (HSR). If the test is positive, you shouldn't take abacavir. If it's negative, you're extremely unlikely to develop HSR.

Hodgkin's disease: A type of lymphoma that is more common in people with HIV but is less common than non-Hodgkin's lymphoma (NHL).

Home test: An HIV blood test that can be performed at home.

HPV: *See* **Human papillomavirus**.

HRA: *See* **High-resolution anoscopy**.

HSR: *See* **Hypersensitivity reaction**.

Human herpesvirus-8: *See* **HHV-8**.

Human immunodeficiency virus: *See* **HIV**.

Human papillomavirus (HPV): A sexually transmitted virus that causes abnormal cells (dysplasia) in the cervix, anus, and mouth, which can lead to cancer if not treated.

Humoral immune system: The part of the immune system that uses antibodies to fight infection. It is less affected by HIV than the cellular immune system.

Hyperlipidemia: An abnormal elevation of lipids (cholesterol and/or triglycerides) in the blood.

Hypersensitivity reaction (HSR): A reaction, often allergic, to a medication or other substance.

Hypogonadism: A deficiency of testosterone, the male sex hormone.

Hypothyroidism: A deficiency in thyroid hormone.

I

Immune activation: A general stimulation of the immune system that can be caused by a variety of infections, including HIV. In the case of HIV, it is thought to cause the decline in CD4 count that occurs with time.

Immune-based therapy: Treatment for HIV designed to affect the immune system and its response to the virus, as opposed to standard antiretroviral therapy, which suppresses the virus itself.

Immune reconstitution inflammatory syndrome (IRIS): A condition that sometimes occurs in people with low CD4 counts who start ART in which the improved immune system reacts to organisms (such as MAC, the TB bacterium, or fungi), causing illness, including fevers, weight loss, swollen lymph nodes, or abscesses.

Immune system: The system in the body that fights infection.

Immunodeficiency (or **immunosuppression**): A state in which the immune system is damaged or impaired, either from birth (congenital immunodeficiency) or acquired, as in HIV.

Indeterminate HIV test: This occurs when the EIA is positive but the Western blot contains some bands that are seen with HIV, though not enough to make a diagnosis. This can occur during the process of seroconversion or it can be found in uninfected people, usually for unclear reasons.

Induced sputum: A test used to diagnose PCP or tuberculosis in which patients inhale a saline mist that makes them cough deeply. The sputum specimen is then sent to the lab for analysis. Also called "sputum induction."

Influenza ("flu"): A viral infection caused by influenza virus that causes fever, muscle aches, respiratory symptoms, and gastrointestinal symptoms during winter months and should be prevented by vaccination in the fall. A bad cold is not the flu.

INH: *See* **Isoniazid**.

Insulin resistance: A condition in which the body cannot respond to insulin as well as it should. This applies both to insulin naturally produced by the pancreas and insulin injected as medication. Can lead to high blood sugar or diabetes.

Integrase: A viral enzyme that allows integration (insertion) of viral DNA into human DNA.

Integrase inhibitor: An antiretroviral drug that blocks the integration process.

Integration: The insertion of viral DNA into human DNA in the nucleus of the cell.

Interferon: An injectable medication used in the past to treat hepatitis C and sometimes hepatitis B.

Interferon-gamma releasing assay (IGRA): A blood test used to detect latent infection with the TB bacterium as an alternative to a tuberculin skin test. *QuantiFERON-TB Gold* is the most commonly used IGRA.

IRIS: *See* **Immune reconstitution inflammatory syndrome**.

Isosporiasis: A disease caused by the parasite *Isospora belli*, which causes chronic diarrhea in people with low CD4 counts. Uncommon in the United States and other developed countries.

Isoniazid (INH): A drug used to treat or prevent tuberculosis.

J

JC virus: The cause of progressive multifocal leukoencephalopathy (PML).

K

Kaposi's sarcoma (KS): A tumor caused by a virus that is more common in people with HIV, especially gay men. Although it usually affects the skin, KS can also affect other parts of the body, including the gastrointestinal tract and lungs.

Kaposi's sarcoma–associated herpesvirus (KSHV): *See* **HHV-8**.

Kidney biopsy: A procedure in which a piece of a kidney is removed using a needle inserted through the skin in order to find out the cause of kidney disorders.

Koch's postulates: The four criteria needed to prove that a microbe or organism is the cause of a disease. The postulates are: (1) The organism must be found in all animals suffering from the disease but should not be found in healthy animals; (2) the organism must be isolated from a diseased animal and grown in pure culture; (3) the cultured organism should cause disease when introduced into a healthy animal; and (4) the organism must be reisolated from the experimentally infected animal.

KS: *See* **Kaposi's sarcoma**.

KSHV: *See* **Kaposi's sarcoma–associated herpesvirus**.

L

Lactic acidosis: A dangerous build-up of lactic acid (lactate) in the blood, which can be caused by some antiretroviral drugs and also by other medical conditions.

Latency: The ability of HIV to persist in human cells for the lifetime of an infected individual by inserting its DNA into long-lived reservoir cells.

Latency-reversing agents: Drugs being studied in experimental cure strategies that activate HIV-infected resting CD4 cells in order to eliminate the latent reservoir (*see* **Shock and kill**).

Leucovorin (or **folinic acid**): A drug used to prevent bone marrow toxicity due to pyrimethamine.

Leukopenia: A decrease in the number of white blood cells found in blood.

LGV: *See* **Lymphogranuloma venereum**.

Life cycle: In HIV, the stages that the virus goes through, starting with its entry into human cells and ending with its replication and the release of new virus particles into the blood.

Lipid panel: A blood test that measures lipid levels in your blood (cholesterol and fats).

Lipoatrophy: Loss of subcutaneous fat (fat under the skin) in the legs, arms, buttocks, and face, caused by some nucleoside analog reverse transcriptase inhibitors (NRTIs).

Lipodystrophy: A general term for changes in body shape and fat distribution caused by some antiretroviral agents. Can include lipoatrophy, fat accumulation, or both.

Lipohypertrophy: *See* **Fat accumulation**.

Listeria: A foodborne bacterium that can cause meningitis and other infections. Although not common, the risk for acquiring *Listeria* is higher in people with HIV.

Liver cancer: *See* **Hepatocellular carcinoma**.

Liver enzymes: *See* **Transaminases**.

Liver toxicity (or **hepatotoxicity**): Damage to the liver caused by medications.

Living will: A legal document that allows you to state which medical procedures and life-sustaining measures you would want if you were no longer able to make decisions for yourself.

Log (logarithm): Another way of expressing viral load results. A viral load of 100,000 is a viral load of five logs; 10,000 is four logs; 1,000 is three logs. A tenfold change in viral load is a one-log change. For example, a drop in viral load from 100,000 to 1,000 is a "two-log drop."

Lumbar puncture: *See* **Spinal tap**.

Lymph nodes: Structures of the human body that are part of the immune system, acting as filters that collect and destroy bacteria and viruses.

Lymphadenopathy: Swollen or enlarged lymph nodes ("glands").

Lymphocyte: A type of infection-fighting white blood cell. CD4 cells are a type of lymphocyte.

Lymphogranuloma venereum (LGV): A sexually transmitted infection caused by *Chlamydia*.

M

MAC: *See* **Mycobacterium avium complex**.

MAI: *See* **Mycobacterium avium complex**.

Medicaid: An insurance program funded by the federal and state governments that provides coverage for medical care to low-income, uninsured people.

Meningitis: An infection or inflammation of the spinal fluid and the lining of the spinal cord.

Meningococcal vaccine: A vaccine that prevents meningococcal disease.

Meningococcus: The bacteria that causes meningococcal disease and meningitis, a serious, potentially life-threatening infection.

Methicillin-resistant *Staphylococcus aureus* (MRSA): A drug-resistant bacterium that traditionally caused serious illness in seriously ill, hospitalized patients but that has recently become a common cause of skin disease, including abscesses (community-acquired MRSA).

Microsporidia: A variety of opportunistic parasites that cause chronic diarrhea in people with low CD4 counts.

Migraine headache: A severe headache, often on one side of the head, sometimes accompanied by visual changes or nausea.

Molluscum contagiosum: Flesh-colored bumps or protuberances on the skin that are caused by a poxvirus and can be sexually transmitted.

Mother-to-child transmission: Transmission of HIV from mother to infant during late pregnancy, labor, or breastfeeding.

MRSA: *See* **Methicillin-resistant Staphylococcus aureus**.

Mucosal cells: Cells that line the internal organs and body orifices, such as the mouth, nostrils, anus, and genital area.

Mutation: Changes in the normal genetic makeup of an organism due to a mistake that occurs during reproduction. In the case of HIV, some mutations can cause resistance, allowing the virus to replicate in the presence of antiretroviral drugs.

Mycobacterium avium complex (MAC): A bacterium related to tuberculosis that causes disease in people with advanced HIV disease, including fever, night sweats, weight loss, diarrhea, liver disease, abdominal pain, and anemia. Also known as *Mycobacterium avium intracellulare* (MAI).

Myelitis: Infection or inflammation of the spinal cord.

Myopathy: An inflammation of muscles causing muscle pain and weakness, sometimes seen with acute retroviral syndrome, high-dose zidovudine, or statin drugs used to lower cholesterol.

N

National Institutes of Health (NIH): An agency of the federal government (under the U.S. Department of Health and Human Services) responsible for conducting and funding medical research.

Nephropathy, HIV-associated (HIVAN): A disease of the kidneys caused by HIV. It is seen primarily in black patients.

Neuropathy (or **peripheral neuropathy**): Damage to the nerves resulting in numbness or burning pain, usually in the feet or legs. Can be caused by HIV, some antiretroviral drugs, or other conditions.

Neuropsychological testing: A series of tests, usually performed by a psychologist or neurologist, to assess memory and thinking skills. Can be used to diagnose dementia or to determine whether someone has depression or dementia.

NHL: *See* **Non-Hodgkin's lymphoma**.

NIH: *See* **National Institutes of Health**.

NNRTIs: *See* **Non-nucleoside reverse transcriptase inhibitors**.

Non-Hodgkin's lymphoma (NHL): The most common type of lymphoma in people with HIV.

Non-nucleoside reverse transcriptase inhibitors (NNRTIs): A class of antiretroviral drugs that blocks reverse transcription of viral RNA into DNA by interfering with the activity of reverse transcriptase.

Non-steroidal anti-inflammatory drugs (NSAIDs): Drugs that are commonly used to suppress inflammation and treat pain. Some are available without a prescription.

NRTIs: *See* **Nucleoside analog reverse transcriptase inhibitors**.

NSAIDs: *See* **Non-steroidal anti-inflammatory drugs**.

Nucleoside analog reverse transcriptase inhibitors (or **NRTIs,** or **"nukes"**): A class of antiretroviral drugs that blocks reverse transcription of viral RNA into DNA by mimicking nucleosides, the normal building blocks of DNA.

"Nukes": *See* **Nucleoside analog reverse transcriptase inhibitors**.

Nystatin: An antifungal mouth rinse used to treat thrush.

O

Odynophagia: Painful swallowing.

OI: *See* **Opportunistic infections**.

Opportunistic infections (OIs): Infections that takes advantage of immunodeficiency. Some opportunistic infections occur *only* in people who are immunosuppressed; others can occur in anyone but are more severe or progressive with immunosuppression.

Oral hairy leukoplakia (OHL): Painless white plaques, or "stripes," on the sides of the tongue caused by Epstein-Barr virus.

Oropharyngeal candidiasis: *Candida* (yeast) infection involving the mouth and throat, including thrush, angular cheilitis, and erythematous candidiasis.

Osteonecrosis: Damage to bones at the large joints (*see* **Avascular necrosis**).

Osteopenia: Loss of bone density ("thinning of the bones").

Osteoporosis: Severe osteopenia, which can lead to bone fractures.

P

Pancreas: An organ in the abdomen that makes insulin and enzymes that help digest food.

Pancreatitis: Inflammation of the pancreas, resulting in abdominal pain, loss of appetite, nausea, and vomiting. Can be fatal.

Pandemic: A global epidemic.

Pan-genotypic: Those hepatitis C treatments that work against all genotypes.

Pap smear: A diagnostic test used to look for cervical dysplasia and cervical cancer. Now also being used to diagnose anal dysplasia (*see* **Anal Pap smear**).

Pathogen: An infectious organism (bacterium, virus, fungus, or parasite) that causes disease.

PCNSL: *See* **Primary central nervous system lymphoma**.

PCP: Used to stand for *Pneumocystis carinii* pneumonia, one of the most common OIs in an HIV-positive patient. It now stands for *Pneumocystis pneumonia*, because of the change in the species name (*see* ***Pneumocystis***).

PCR: *See* **Polymerase chain reaction**.

Peliosis hepatis: An uncommon bacterial liver infection caused by *Bartonella*.

Pelvic inflammatory disease (PID): A serious infection of the uterus and fallopian tubes usually caused by sexually transmitted infections, especially gonorrhea and chlamydia.

Pentamidine: A drug used to treat PCP. Aerosolized pentamidine is sometimes used as an inhaled mist to prevent PCP.

Peripheral neuropathy: *See* **Neuropathy**.

Pharynx: Throat.

Persistent low-level viremia: Viral load that is repeatedly detectable between 20 and 200 copies despite being on antiretroviral threapy.

Phenotype test: A type of resistance test that measures the ability of the virus to replicate in varying concentrations of antiretroviral drugs.

PID: *See* **Pelvic inflammatory disease**.

Plasma HIV RNA: *See* **Viral load**.

Platelets: Blood cells that help blood clot. A low platelet count, which can sometimes occur due to HIV, can result in easy bleeding or bruising.

PML: *See* **Progressive multifocal leukoencephalopathy**.

Pneumococcal vaccine: A vaccine (*Prevnar 13, Pneumovax*) recommended for HIV-positive adults to prevent pneumonia caused by pneumococcus.

Pneumococcus: The common name for *Streptococcus pneumoniae*, a frequent cause of bacterial pneumonia.

Pneumocystis: A fungus (*Pneumocystis jiroveci*) that is a common cause of pneumonia (PCP) in people with HIV.

Pneumonia: An infection of the air spaces of the lungs, which can be caused by a variety of infectious organisms.

Polymerase chain reaction (PCR): A laboratory technique used to detect or quantify the DNA or RNA of an infectious organism for diagnostic purposes.

PPD: *See* **Tuberculin skin test**.

Pre-exposure prophylaxis (PrEP): A form of HIV prevention in which antiretroviral medications are taken by HIV-negative individuals to prevent infection.

PrEP: *See* **Pre-exposure prophylaxis**.

Primary central nervous system lymphoma (PCNSL): A lymphoma involving the brain, seen only in people with advanced HIV disease.

Primary HIV: The stage of HIV that occurs shortly after infection. At this stage, the viral load is very high but antibody tests may be negative or indeterminate. People often have symptoms during this stage (*see* **Acute retroviral syndrome**).

Proctitis: Infection or inflammation of the rectum.

Progressive multifocal leukoencephalopathy (PML): An infection of the brain caused by JC virus, which results in progressive neurologic deterioration.

Prophylaxis: Prevention, usually applied to the use of medications taken to prevent opportunistic infections or to keep them from coming back after they've been treated.

Protease: A viral enzyme that cuts large viral proteins into smaller proteins, which are then used to create new virus particles. A protease inhibitor (PI) is an antiretroviral drug that blocks this process.

Prurigo nodularis: A condition characterized by itchy bumps on the skin, seen more commonly in people with HIV.

Psoriasis: A skin condition that results in dry, scaly, itchy plaques on the skin that can get worse with immunosuppression due to HIV.

Purified protein derivative (PPD): *See* **Tuberculin skin test**.

Pyrimethamine: A drug used to treat or prevent PCP or toxoplasmosis.

Q

QuantiFERON-TB Gold: The most commonly used interferon-gamma releasing assay (IGRA), a blood test for latent tuberculosis infection.

R

R5 virus: HIV that enters the CD4 cell using the CCR5 coreceptor. This type of virus can be treated with CCR5 inhibitors (*see* **Coreceptors**).

Radiculitis (radiculopathy): Infection or inflammation of the nerves that emerge from the spinal cord.

Rapid tests: HIV tests that provide an answer within a few minutes, using either blood or saliva. Positive tests must be confirmed with standard serologies.

Reactive airways: *See* **Bronchospasm**.

Recombinant strains: Strains of HIV that are combinations of two or more other strains.

Red blood cell (RBC): Blood cells that carry oxygen to the organs of the body. If you don't have enough RBCs, you're anemic.

Regimen: A combination of antiretroviral drugs.

Relapse: The return of an illness or disease, usually in someone with a chronic condition.

Replication: The reproduction or multiplication of an organism, including HIV. The replication of HIV is a complex, multi-step process involving infection of a human cell and use of both viral enzymes and human cellular machinery to create new virus particles, which are then released and can infect new cells.

Reservoir: Long-lived human cells that can be infected by HIV, allowing it to persist (remain latent) for the lifetime of the individual. Resting CD4 cells are the best known example, but there are other reservoirs in the human body.

Resistance: The ability of the virus to replicate despite the presence of antiretroviral medications.

Resistance test: A blood test (either a genotype or phenotype) that looks for HIV that is resistant to antiretroviral medications.

Resting CD4 cells: CD4 cells that live a long time and can harbor HIV DNA, which can't be affected by antiretroviral therapy because the cell is not replicating, and thus are an important reservoir of latent HIV.

Retinitis: An infection of the retina (the interior surface of the back of the eye), which can lead to blindness if not treated. Most often caused by CMV.

Retrovirus: A virus that contains RNA and that can turn RNA into DNA through reverse transcription using viral enzymes. (*See* **Reverse transcription**.) HIV is a retrovirus.

Reverse transcriptase (RT): An enzyme contained within the HIV virus that can turn viral RNA into DNA so it can be inserted into the DNA of human cells. A reverse transcriptase inhibitor blocks this process.

Reverse transcription: The conversion of viral RNA into DNA by reverse transcriptase. (Normal transcription involves the conversion of DNA into RNA.)

Rifabutin: A drug used to treat or prevent MAC. It is also used as an alternative to rifampin to treat tuberculosis.

Rifampin: A drug used to treat tuberculosis and some other bacterial infections.

RNA: Ribonucleic acid, the genetic material of the HIV virus. Viral RNA gets turned into DNA by reverse transcriptase, and the viral DNA then gets inserted into the DNA of human cells. DNA is later transcribed back into RNA, which in turn gets translated into the proteins that are used to make new virus particles.

RT: *See* **Reverse transcriptase**.

Ryan White Care Act: A government-funded program that provides money on a state or local level to provide care for uninsured people with HIV.

S

Salmonella: A group of bacteria that can cause severe diarrhea, fever, and bloodstream infections.

Scabies: An itchy skin condition caused by a mite that burrows under the skin and can be spread to others by close contact.

Seborrheic dermatitis: A common skin condition causing flakiness on the face, especially around the eyebrows and in the folds on the cheeks.

Septra: *See* **Trimethoprim-sulfamethoxazole**.

Seroconversion: The process of developing an antibody to an infectious agent. In the case of HIV, it occurs shortly after primary infection.

Serologies: Blood tests that measure antibodies or antigens to look for evidence of a disease.

Sexually transmitted infections (STIs): Infections transmitted from person to person through sexual activity. Also called sexually transmitted diseases (STDs).

Shingles (or **herpes zoster**): A painful, blistering rash, usually occurring in a linear band on one side of the body, caused by reactivation of the chickenpox virus (varicella-zoster virus, VZV).

Shock and kill: An experimental cure strategy in which HIV-infected resting CD4 cells are first activated by latency-reversing agents, allowing the virus to be treated with antiretroviral therapy.

Side effects: Undesirable effects of a medication or treatment that are noticeable to the person being treated (*see* **Toxicity**).

Sinus headache: A headache caused by congestion of the sinuses (*see* **Sinusitis**).

Sinusitis: An infection of the sinuses, which are air spaces in the head connected to the nasal passages.

Social Security Disability Insurance (SSDI): A monthly Social Security benefit for disabled people who have worked in the past and have paid a minimum amount of Social Security taxes.

Sperm washing: A technique in which sperm are separated from semen to lower the risk of HIV transmission to a woman during conception.

Spinal tap (or lumbar puncture): A procedure in which a needle is inserted into the back between the vertebrae to collect a sample of cerebrospinal fluid (CSF) to diagnose meningitis. (Not as bad as it sounds.)

SSDI: *See* **Social Security Disability Insurance**.

SSI: *See* **Supplemental Security Income**.

Statins: The common name for HMG CoA reductase inhibitors, drugs that lower cholesterol.

STIs: *See* **Sexually transmitted infections**.

Strain: In the case of HIV, a type of virus, as in "drug-resistant strain."

Strep throat: The common term for *streptococcal pharyngitis*, a bacterial infection of the throat caused by group A beta-hemolytic *Streptococcus*.

Structured treatment interruption: An old term for an interruption in therapy that was approved by the provider.

Subcutaneous fat: Fat found under the skin.

Subtypes: In the case of HIV, groups of related viruses, also called "clades" or "sub-clades." Most HIV-positive people in the United States are infected with subtype B, but there are many other subtypes throughout the world.

Superinfection: Reinfection with a new strain of HIV in someone who has already been infected.

Supplemental Security Income (SSI): A federal cash assistance program designed to help the aged, blind, and disabled who have little or no income to pay for basic necessities.

Symptomatic HIV: A stage of HIV in which people have symptoms caused by HIV, such as weight loss, diarrhea, or thrush, but have not yet developed an AIDS indicator condition.

Syndrome: A collection of signs or symptoms that frequently occur together but that may or may not be caused by a single disease. AIDS was referred to as a syndrome before its cause, HIV, had been discovered.

Syphilis: A sexually transmitted infection caused by *Treponema pallidum*, a bacterium, that can cause anal, genital, or mouth lesions (primary syphilis); fever, rash, and hepatitis (secondary syphilis); or infection of the brain, spinal fluid, eyes, or ears (neurosyphilis). It can also be dormant, causing no symptoms (latent syphilis).

T

T-helper cell: *See* **CD4 cell**.

T-suppressor cells: *See* **CD8 cells**.

TB: *See* **Tuberculosis**.

Tdap: *See* **Tetanus toxoid**.

Tension headache: A headache caused by muscle tension.

Testosterone: The male sex hormone, which can be low in some HIV-positive men (*see* **Hypogonadism**).

Tetanus toxoid (dT or Tdap): A combination vaccine that should be received every 10 years for adults, regardless of HIV status. Tdap (a combination tetanus, diphtheria, pertussis vaccine) should be given once.

Therapeutic vaccine: A vaccine given to treat an existing infection by stimulating the immune system to fight it.

Thrombocytopenia: A disorder in which there is an abnormally low number of platelets in the blood.

Thrush: Oral candidiasis, a yeast infection involving the mouth presenting with white/yellow curd-like plaques on the palate, gums, or the back of the throat.

TMP-SMX: A combination of two antibiotic drugs used to treat a wide variety of bacterial infections (*see* **Trimethoprim-sulfamethoxazole**).

Toxicity: Damage to the body caused by a drug or other substance.

Toxoplasma: A parasite (*Toxoplasma gondii*) that causes brain lesions (encephalitis) in people with HIV.

Toxoplasmosis: Disease caused by the parasite, *Toxoplasma gondii*.

Transaminases (or liver enzymes): Blood tests used to look for damage to the liver.

Transcription: The process of turning DNA into RNA.

Treatment interruption: Stopping antiretroviral therapy. No longer in vogue.

Triglycerides: Fats that are ingested in the form of vegetable oils and animal fats.

Trimethoprim-sulfamethoxazole (TMP-SMX, cotrimoxazole, *Bactrim, Septra*): An antibiotic used to treat or prevent PCP and to prevent toxoplasmosis.

Tropism assay: A blood test used to find out whether your virus enters the CD4 cell using the CCR5 coreceptor (R5 virus) or the CXCR4 coreceptor (X4 virus). This test is necessary before taking a CCR5 inhibitor, which should only be used with R5 virus.

Tuberculin skin test (TST, or purified protein derivative [PPD]): A skin test used to look for evidence of past exposure to *Mycobacterium tuberculosis*, the bacterium that causes tuberculosis. The most common form of TST is the PPD (purified protein derivative).

Tuberculosis (TB): A bacterial disease caused by *Mycobacterium tuberculosis*. TB most often causes lung disease but can affect any part of the body.

Typhoid vaccine: A vaccine to prevent typhoid fever, a bacterial infection of the blood caused by *Salmonella typhi*, sometimes acquired by travelers to developing countries.

U

Undetectable: A term used to describe a viral load that is too low to be measured by a viral load test. An undetectable viral load is below 20 with the most commonly used test.

Urinalysis: A standard lab test that looks for evidence of protein, sugar, blood, and infection in the urine.

V

Vaccine (vaccination): A substance that is given, usually by injection, but sometimes by mouth or by nasal spray, to stimulate the immune system to make antibodies against a bacterial or viral pathogen.

Vaginitis: Infection or inflammation of the vagina.

Valacyclovir: A drug used to treat herpes simplex and varicella-zoster virus.

Varicella-zoster virus: The virus that causes chickenpox (primary varicella) and shingles (herpes zoster).

Viral load (or **plasma HIV RNA**): A lab test that measures the amount of HIV virus in the plasma (blood), expressed as "copies per milliliter." The viral load predicts the rate of progression to AIDS. It is the most important test for measuring the effectiveness of ART and also helps determine the need for treatment.

Virions: Single virus particles.

Virus: A microscopic organism composed of genetic material (DNA or RNA) inside a protein coat.

Visceral fat: Fat present inside the abdomen, around the internal organs, rather than under the skin.

W

WB: *See* **Western blot**.

WBC: *See* **White blood cell**.

Western blot (WB): Traditionally, the confirmatory test used to diagnose HIV in people who tested positive for HIV antibodies by ELISA.

White blood cell (WBC): A type of blood cell that helps fight infection. CD4 cells are a type of lymphocyte, which is a type of white blood cell.

Wild-type virus: The strain of HIV that occurs "in the wild"—without the presence of antiretroviral drugs that could select for mutations. Generally a non-mutant, drug-sensitive virus.

Window period: The period between infection and formation of antibodies leading to a positive HIV test (serology).

X

X4 (or dual/mixed [D/M]) virus: HIV that enters the CD4 cell using the CXCR4 coreceptor. X4 virus cannot be treated with CCR5 inhibitors (*see* **Coreceptors**).

Y

Yeast: A group of microorganisms that can sometimes cause human infections, ranging from minor (oral thrush, vaginitis) to severe (cryptococcal meningitis). All yeasts are fungi.

Yellow fever: A serious disease caused by yellow fever virus, which is transmitted by mosquitoes and sometimes acquired by travelers to parts of Africa or Latin America.

Index